LEPROSY

A Reference Guide for Medical Practitioners, Programme Managers and Leprosy Workers

About the Author

DR. R.S. MISRA, M.B.B.S., M.D., D.D., is at present Consultant Dermato-Venereologist and Leprologist, and Head of the Department of Dermatology, Leprology and Regional STD Teaching, Training and Research Centre, Safdarjang Hospital, Government of India, New Delhi. He is a clinician of long standing with keen interest in research in infective dermatoses, leprosy and STDs. Dr. Misra has more than 70 research papers published in national and international journals to his credit. He had been teacher of undergraduate medical students in the University College of Medical Sciences and is presently Supervisor of Post-graduate students of Dermatology and Venereology of the Delhi University.

He had been a long-time advocate of a uniform multiple-drug therapy implementation, irrespective of endemicity of the disease in the region — a point which is now being appreciated and implemented by the National Leprosy Eradication Programme in India. Dr. Misra is an active health-educationist, member of expert committees of various organisations and programme implementation committees concerned with the welfare programmes for leprosy affected patients.

LEPROSY

A Reference Guide for Medical Practitioners, Programme Managers and Leprosy Workers

Dr. R.S. Misra, MD., D.D.

Consultant, Dermato-Venereologist and Leprologist, and
Head, Department of Dermatology, Leprology and
Regional STD Teaching, Training and Research Centre
Safdarjang Hospital, Government of India, New Delhi

CONCEPT PUBLISHING COMPANY, NEW DELHI 110059

ISBN 81-7022-472-1

First Published 1993

Published and Printed by
Ashok Kumar Mittal
Concept Publishing Company
A/15-16, Commercial Block, Mohan Garden
NEW DELHI-110059 (India)

Lasertypeset by
Microtech Advance Printing Systems (Pvt.) Ltd.
H-13, Bali Nagar
NEW DELHI-110015

FOREWORD

Leprosy control in India and elsewhere is passing through an extremely interesting phase as has been the case during the past ten to twelve years. For the first time, the public health aspects of the disease are given a high priority with clear goals for attaining elimination of the disease as a public health problem in a given period of time. Leprosy workers with varying backgrounds have been able to come together to fight for the common cause of leprosy and set an example to workers in other fields of health. The phenomenal success of leprosy control in several parts of India, thanks to widespread implementation of multidrug therapy (MDT), has indeed encouraged several countries to intensify their efforts in leprosy control. Notwithstanding the progress made and the optimistic outlook, some aspects of the disease such as disabilities among existing and cured patients continue to pose significant problems to leprosy endemic communities. In the long run, however, disability problems in leprosy are expected to diminish together with steady decreases in prevalence and incidence of the disease itself.

Several problems relating to leprosy in India deserve special attention including the problem of how to handle leprosy control in low endemic areas, and how to motivate and train general health workers including physicians in leprosy. Discussions of such topics in medical colleges and other sectors traditionally not carrying out leprosy work will be a useful step to widen their interest in leprosy work and to enable them to participate in leprosy control.

This publication by Dr. R.S. Misra, is a very interesting compilation of reference material produced by various governmental and non-governmental bodies as well as well written contributions on several technical aspects of leprosy, and is likely to be of great value to relevant leprosy workers.

Dr. S.K. Noordeen
Chief Medical Officer, Leprosy Unit
Division of Control of Tropical Diseases
World Health Organization
CH-1211 Geneva 27
Switzerland

PREFACE

Leprosy situation has considerably improved during the last decade. The developments in the fields of therapeutics, immunology and biotechnology has changed the face of leprosy from near hopeless casting its social and psychological pall to one with that of amenability to treatment in a short period of time without stigmatising deformities and ulcers. The wealth of knowledge and available expertise in the field has made it possible to deal with leprosy effectively leading to its eradication if adequate financial resources are made available for the managerial and organisational infrastructure to accomplish the job.

Interactions with the faculty and participants of a workshop on Multi-drug Therapy of Leprosy in Low-endemic Areas of India, served as a nucleus for developing the basics into the present work. In the text the leprosy situation in various world regions is exhaustively reviewed, attention has been focused on problems encountered during management of the disease by the medical and paramedical personnel under the field conditions, and solutions are suggested. A co-ordinated and concerted line of action on the part of various agencies involved in the Leprosy Eradication Programme has been put forth to handle the situation. The knowledge available in the fields of therapeutics, IEC, immunology and biotechnology, etc., its efficacy and application so far and future prospects are discussed in order to evolve a suitable strategy for eradication of leprosy from all the areas — be they hyperendemic or comparatively low in endemicity of the disease.

This presentation would have more than achieved its purpose if it is found useful by the large number of medical and paramedical workers involved in the gigantic task of eradication of leprosy and give them much sought for information at one place to deal with the latest developments in the field.

Acknowledgements

I gratefully acknowledge the encouragement given by Dr. A.K. Mukherjee, Director General of Health Services, Government of India, from time to time to pursue my interest in this field. I am also thankful to Dr. S.K. Noordeen, Chief Medical Officer, Leprosy Unit, World Health Organisation, who acceded to my request of writing Foreword to the volume. I acknowledge and appreciate the help given by Dr. B.N. Mittal, Deputy Director General of Health Services and Dr. N.S. Dharmshaktu, Assistant Director General Health Services in Leprosy Division of DGHS for making available to me reports and relevant information about the Programme in India. I put on record my deep sense of appreciation to all the contributors to the text who despite their many pressing engagements submitted the manuscripts well in time to make this volume comprehensive. I am thankful to all my patients who are a constant source of inspiration to delve into the problem deeply and think of newer innovations.

I appreciate the efforts of Ms Geeta Sabharwal for typing out the script neatly. My thanks are also due to Shri Ashok Kumar Mittal, Concept Publishing Company, New Delhi for undertaking the publication on priority basis and coping with the tedious process of handling the manuscript overcoming the various odds. Last but not the least, I am thankful to my wife, Dr. Nisha Misra, for putting up with my idiosyncracies in the matter of collecting the literature and writing the text.

January 1993 R.S. MISRA

CONTENTS

PART III
INDIAN SCENARIO

PART IV
PROBLEMS IN LEPROSY MANAGEMENT

PART V
FACETS OF LEPROSY ERADICATION

Appendices

National Leprosy Eradication Programme (NLEP)

Implementation of NLEP

LIST OF TABLES

LIST OF FIGURES

ABBREVIATIONS COMMONLY USED AND THEIR CONNOTATIONS

AFB	–	Acid Fast Bacilli
AIR	–	All India Radio
BB	–	Pure Borderline
BI	–	Bacteriological Index
BL	–	Borderline Lepromatous
BT	–	Borderline Tuberculoid
CDMO	–	Chief District Medical Officer
CHC	–	Community Health Centre
CHG	–	Community Health Guide
DD	–	Doordarshan (Hindi equivalent of Television)
DDP	–	Drug Distribution Point
DDS	–	Dapsone
DGHS	–	Director General of Health Services
DHO	–	District Health Officer
DHS	–	Director of Health Services
DLO	–	District Leprosy Officer
ENL	–	Erythema Nodosum Leprosum
FDT	–	Fixed Duration Therapy
G.I. Tract	–	Gastro Intestinal Tract
HE	–	Health Education or Health Educator
HG	–	Health Guide
HS	–	Health Supervisor
I	–	Indeterminate
IAL	–	Indian Association of Leprologists
IT	–	Intensive Treatment
L	–	Lepromatous
L&N	–	Doubtful cases which could be Lepromatous or Non-Lepromatous
LCU	–	Leprosy Control Unit
LL	–	Lepromatous Leprosy
MA	–	Maculo Anaesthetic

MB – Multi Bacillary
MCR – Micro Cellular Rubber
MDT – Multi-drug therapy
M. Leprae – Mycobacterium Leprae
MO – Medical Officer
MPW – Multi Purpose Worker
N – Non-lepromatous
N?L – Borderline Leprosy
NLCP – National Leprosy Control Programme
NLEP – National Leprosy Eradication Programme
NMA – Non Medical Assistant
NMS – Non Medical Supervisor
NSS – National Social Service
P – Pure Neuritic
PB – Pauci Bacillary
PHC – Primary Health Centre
PH Care – Primary Health Care
PMS – Para Medical Supervisor
PMW – Para Medical Worker
POL – Petrol, Oil, Lubricants
RFT – Release From Treatment
RMP – Registered Medical Practitioner
SC – Sub Centre
SET – Survey, Education and Treatment Centre
SHC – Subsidiary Health Centre
SHE – Senior Health Educator
SHEB – State Health Education Bureau
SLO – State Leprosy Officer
SS – School Survey
T – Tuberculoid
THW – Temporary Hospitalisation Ward
ULC – Urban Leprosy Centre
UNICEF – United Nations Children's Fund
WHO – World Health Organisation
ZLO – Zonal Leprosy Officer

LIST OF CONTRIBUTORS

1. **Dr. A.C. McDougall,** MD (Edin), FRCP (London), MRCP (Edin)
Formerly Consultant in Clinical Investigation (Leprosy)
Department of Dermatology, The Slade Hospital,
Headington, Oxford, OX37JH, ENGLAND

2. **Dr. Maria da Graça Cunha**
Director
Instituto de Dermatologia Tropical
"Alfredo da Matta"
Manus, Amazone, BRAZIL

3. **Dr. Gerson Oliveira Penna**
Instituto de Dermatologia Tropical
"Alfredo da Matta"
Manus, Amazonas, BRAZIL

4. **Dr. Gerson Fernando Mendes**
Instituto de Dermatologia Tropical
"Alfredo da Matta"
Manus, Amazonas, BRAZIL

5. **Dr. Maria da Fatima Maroja**
c/o Director
Instituto de Dermatologia Tropical
"Alfredo da Matta"
Manus, Amazonas, BRAZIL

6. **Dr. R. Ganapati,** MBBS, DDV
Director
Bombay Leprosy Project
6/27, Amar Bhuvan, Sion (East)
Bombay-400022, INDIA

7. **Dr. Kiran Katoch,** MD
Assistant Director and Head Medical Unit I
Central JALMA Institute for Leprosy,
PO Box 31, Taj Ganj
Agra-282001, INDIA

8. **Dr. G. Ramu,** MD
Consultant
Sacred Heart Leprosy Centre and
Voluntary Health Services Leprosy Control Project,
Sakthinagar
1705, 3E, Pioneer Complex
Avinasi Road,
Coimbatore-641018, INDIA

9. **Dr. B.K. Girdhar,** MD
Deputy Director (Clinical)
Central JALMA Institute for Leprosy,
PO Box 31, Taj Ganj
Agra-282001, INDIA

10. **Dr. V.N. Bhatia,** MD
Serologist to the Government of India
3 Kyd Street
Calcutta-700016, INDIA

11. **Dr. Ernest P. Fritschi,** MB, FRCS (Edin), D.Orth.
Former Director and Consultant Surgeon
Schieffelin Leprosy Research and Training Centre
Karigiri, North Arcot District
Tamil Nadu-632106, INDIA

12. **Dr. Navnit K. Sharma,** MD
Professor and Head
Department of Dermato-Venereology
Lala Lajpat Rai Memorial Medical College
Meerut, INDIA

13. **Dr. B.M.S. Bedi,** MD, FAMS, FCAI
    Director-Professor and Head
    Department of Dermatology and STD
    Maulana Azad Medical College
    New Delhi-110002, INDIA

14. **Dr. A.B. Hiramani,** Ph.D.
    Deputy Director (Research)
    Central Health Education Bureau
    Government of India
    Kotla Road
    New Delhi-110002, INDIA

15. **Dr. Atul C. Shah**, MS, MNAMS
    Reconstructive Surgeon
    Project Director
    Comprehensive Leprosy Care Project
    Honorary Assistant Surgeon of Plastic Surgery
    Grant Medical College and Sir J.J. Group of Hospital
    Byculla
    Bombay-400008, INDIA

16. **Dr. Thomas Abraham**
    Technical Adviser
    German Leprosy Relief Association
    4, Gajapathi Street
    Shenoynagar
    Madras-600030, INDIA

17. **Dr. Rama Mukherjee**, PhD
    Head, Microbiology Division
    National Institute of Immunology
    Shahid Jeet Singh Marg
    New Delhi-110067, INDIA

1

LEPROSY AT A TURNING POINT

R.S. MISRA

Gerhard Armauer Hansen (1841-1912) of Norway in 1873 discovered Mycobacterium leprae as the first microbial pathogen responsible for infecting man, dismantling the earlier hereditary theory for the causation of leprosy. M. leprae is an obligatory intracellular parasite with a special affinity for Schwan cells and cells of the reticulo-endothalial system. Till date the organism has defied all attempts of 'in-vitro' culture in laboratory, unlike, many other organisms discovered much after, thus posing a big obstacle in devising effective control measures to eradicate leprosy. Development of animal models, viz., Shepherd's mouse-foot-pad and nine-banded armadillo (*dasypus movemcinctus*) have helped in quantitative bacteriological studies.

Till the early decades of the present century the leprosy patient had remained an object of extreme contempt and social and economic ostracisation. The false religio-social correlation with sins of present or past births further made the plight of leprosy sufferer difficult. To overcome this injustice meted out to these unfortunate ones some missionaries took courageous steps to look after them and establish 'leprosoria' for their care, but the same step became counter-productive and a cause for dehabilitation of the leprosy patient and for perpetuating and strengthening the social stigma against the disease.

The problem of leprosy is three faceted: (i) medical, (ii) public health, and (iii) socio-economic. For the success of any control programme all the activities, required for success of the 'total leprosy control', have to work in close unison.

The most important factor in planning for a disease, such as, leprosy is to find out the exact magnitude of the problem. In India, in this direction, the first steps of finding out information about the rough distribution in the country through leprosy surveys in randomly selected areas in the various parts of each State were taken up by the Indian Council of the British Empire Association, which after Independence of the country in 1947 was named Hind Kusht Nivaran Sangh (Indian Leprosy Association). To conduct the surveys, All India Survey Party was organised which worked through PTS Centres (P=propaganda-publicity, T=treatment, and S=surveys). Since 1955 the leprosy control has been taken up as a thrust area under the Five-Year Plan activities of the Government of India (Dharmendra, 1985). On the international scene the WHO and UNICEF started helping all countries in which leprosy is creating a serious health problem. The WHO set up a special project 'Research and Training in Tropical Diseases', which included leprosy among other important tropical diseases.

What do We Want to Achieve?

The term 'disease control' describes (on-going) operations at reducing:

(i) the incidence of disease;
(ii) the duration of disease, and consequently the risk of transmission;
(iii) the effects of infection, including both the physical and psychosocial complications; and
(iv) the financial burden to the community.

In disease control, the disease 'agent' is permitted to persist in the community at a level when it ceases to be a public health problem according to the tolerance of the local population. A state of equilibrium becomes established between the disease agent, host and environment and components of the disease process.

Disease Elimination

The term 'elimination' is used to describe interruption of transmission of disease from large geographic regions or areas. Regional elimination is now seen as an important precursor of eradication.

Disease Eradication

The term 'eradication' implies termination of all transmission of infection by extermination of the infectious agent. Eradication is an absolute process, and not a relative goal. It is 'all or none phenomenon'. The word 'eradication' is reserved to cessation of infection and disease from the whole world. To date, small-pox is the only disease that has been eradicated (Park and Park, 1989; *definitions*).

In May 1991, the 44th World Health Assembly (WHA) resolved WHO's commitment to continue to promote the use of all control measures including multi-drug therapy (MDT) together with case-finding in order to attain the *global elimination* (elimination of leprosy as a public health problem is defined as the reduction of prevalence below one case per 10,000 population) of leprosy as a public health problem by the year 2000 (WHA, 1991).

In the present volume an assessment of the current situation with regard to leprosy is made from various points of view – global, regional and highly endemic regions. In this context the total global leprosy situation developing over a period of time all over the world is critically reviewed in the background of numbers, efforts made to contain it and the results obtained. To further see the problem in sharp focus, effort is made to review the situation in greater detail in high endemic leprosy regions of the world, i.e., in regions and countries where the prevalence of leprosy is more than 1/1000 at the moment. In the next phase the situation is reviewed region-wise by experts conversant with the regions and those working in the area. Dr. McDougall (Chapter 4) reviews the leprosy situation in Africa, with regard to disease prevalence, the operational strategies adopted and the results obtained so far. In the Americas, Brazil, is one country, which has very acute leprosy problem. The same is reviewed by Dr. Marie da Graca Cunha, Director, Institute of Tropical Dermatology and Venereology 'Alfredo da Matta', et al (5.1 in Chapter 5). In Brazil itself, in particular State of Amazonas, how the leprosy control programme has worked with relation to MDT and early case-detection is further dealt with in 5.2 in Chapter 5.

India, being the single country with the largest number of patients in the world and having 75 per cent of the patients in the South-East Asian region is dealt with in detail (Chapter 6), because the country had been able to reduce the prevalence of leprosy effectively since the implementation of the MDT in the control programme and because of the high political commitment to eradicate the disease by the year 2000. India is further important for leprologists, epidemiologists and students of medical sciences to observe it with keen interest because of varied prevalence of the disease distributed over the vast geographical areas. The programme, whereas it has succeeded in the high-endemic districts (above 5/1000 prevalence) under the operation of vertical programme, has remained uncovered to a large extent in moderately endemic (2-5/1000 prevalence) and low-endemic (1 or below 1/1000 prevalence) areas due to financial and managerial constraints so far. Therefore, besides discussing the operative methodology, results obtained and inputs put in high-endemic areas, the problem of the moderate and low-endemic areas is also reviewed critically in the following chapters. In this connection the IV Independent Evaluation, conducted under the joint auspices of World Health Organisation and Government of India in December 1991, has come as a great help and many experts, like Dr. R. Ganapati and Dr. Kiran Katoch, et al, who were associated with this gigantic task, have given their frank and forthright opinion on the current state of affairs in the areas which they had chance to visit and to verify the facts with regard to disease control activities and the measures required in future to streamline the programme to make it effective (Chapter 7).

Part IV deals with technical problems faced by clinicians, paramedical workers, laboratory technicians, and programme managers, at the operative level in the field. The problem of distinguishing progression of disease *vis-a-vis* reactions in leprosy in patients under treatment, or reporting for the first time, with or without treatment, to the clinician/paramedical worker is discussed in detail by noted leprologist and clinician of vast experience, Dr. G. Ramu for the benefit of large number of leprosy workers working in this field (Chapter 8). Identification of drug-resistance, *vis-a-vis* progression of disease process is still another area, where at times great expertise and keen observation is needed. These two entities, namely, (i) progression of disease *vis-a-vis* Reaction, and (ii) Drug Resistance, become further important in the context of uneven application of MDT in the field. The points made out by Dr. G. Ramu and Dr. B.K. Girdhar can give important practical tips to the leprosy workers (Chapter 9). Another important area is that of management and monitoring of Bacterial Index (BI) in the context of MDT, because the application of MDT is to be varied between abacillary and multibacillary cases depending on BI positivity. In the various evaluations of the programme in the past, the management of BI has been considered as the weakest link in the chain. This important subject has been dealt with in detail by Dr. V.N. Bhatia, a microbiologist with a long and rich experience in leprosy microbiology research (Chapter 10).

The problem of leprosy to a layman is the problem of deformed, disabled hands and feet and unhealing ulcers. The leprosy is bound to remain a social stigma as long as the individuals afflicted with leprosy are seen with deformities of hands and feet. These can be controlled and prevented to large measure by a vigilant medical officer/paramedical worker, if he is able to recognise the impending event and take necessary corrective measures in time and in case of development of such deformity can provide the minimum basic guidance and support to the patient in the initial stages. Keeping this in view, the subject of field management of disabilities/deformities is dealt with by a renowned leprosy reconstructive surgeon, Dr. Ernest P. Fritschi (Chaper 11).

Part V deals with managerial problems at various levels in the field, because the clever and effective management of the situations are the real thing, which help in effective health care of the patient. Dr. Navnit K. Sharma, Professor of Dermatology and Venereology in a Medical College, discusses the role of specialised centres in leprosy control programme and sums up how the activities of these Centres can coordinate with the peripheral level of health care facilities in the area (Chapter 12).

Dr. B.M.S. Bedi, Professor of Dermatology and Venereology, having long years of experience in both low-endemic and high endemic areas has discussed the problems of monitoring of MDT in endemic and low-endemic areas and has suggested various measures to overcome the difficulties faced in the field (Chapter 13).

Till of late, leprosy was considered as a problem of high prevalence in rural sector only, where the population had not so much of mobility and it was easy to detect the new cases, trace the contacts, and monitor the drug treatment regularly and effectively. Development and expansion of cosmopolitan cities has brought to the fore the fact that the development of slums in the cities, where people have to perforce live in cramped up space and sub-optimal living conditions, has contributed to and worsened the problem of leprosy in these areas. Dr. R. Ganapati, has portrayed the problem of cosmopolitan cities in the context of Leprosy Control Programme and suggested various measures to counteract and overcome the difficulties faced in the urban set-up (Chapter 14). The most important element, be it early case-detection, contact tracing, regularity of MDT, or early detection of complications in the disease, is health education of the patient and of community, including the health personnel responsible for operating the programme. The role of health education for early detection of leprosy is discussed by Dr. A.B. Hiramani, a social scientist (Chapter 15).

The ideal with regard to availability of resources, manpower, etc., is not likely to be available in the developing and under-developed countries for quite some time to come. Then, how are we going to overcome our present pressing health problems, like, leprosy? A via-media needs to be adopted by judicious distribution of resources utilisation of the available health personnel to achieve the maximum possible benefit, to the best of their capacities and talents. With this end in view, and keeping the WHO advocated concept of implementing leprosy control activities through Primary Health Care set-up, the plan for a strategy for Leprosy Eradication Programme in low-endemic areas is presented and discussed (Chapter 16). Dr. R. Mukherjee has reviewed the immunological and biotechnological developments in the last decade. These efforts have resulted in newer vaccines and diagnostic probes. The ongoing research in this field is towards detecting the disease in the subclinical phase, impending nerve damage, etc., which is going to have great bearing in leprosy control programme (Chapter 17). The results of implementation of MDT during the preceding decade as also future scenario of an effective control programme are reviewed in Chapter 18.

The strategy presented envisages the integration of vertical programme and the Primary Health Care set-up, according to the needs of the area and endemicity of the disease in the region, so that there is neither wastage of the resources by way of underutilisation of the facilities, nor lack of resources at the crucial points, where they are needed the most.

'At the end of 1990 . . . world numbers of registered (leprosy) cases not only ceased to rise, but, despite continued intensive case-detection activities in many countries, showed a significant fall over previous years. For the first time . . . multi-drug therapy was being administered to more than half the known patients in the world in over 90 per cent of countries or areas with leprosy. For the first time, it became reasonable to speak of the eventual disappearance of the disease, atleast as a public health problem . . ." (WHO, 1991).

This new found hope has given us encouragement to look at the problem seriously and to muster all our resources in a coordinated manner, without either under-utilising in the areas, where they are needed the most, or wasting them by over-utilisation from where they can be saved and utilised in the most needed sectors. Keeping this in sight, an overview of various methodologies utilised in various regions of the world is taken and critically reviewed and assessed with the aim of finding the best course out. The presentation of the data has also the idea that it will give the scientists, leprologists and students of medicine to interact with each other after understanding the ground realities of the various regions of the world and try to find an agreement with the following statement made by World Health Organisation:

> In the history of leprosy control, 1991 marks a turning point between the past and the future: a turning point that calls for a pause to take stock of what has been achieved and what remains to be done (WHO, 1991).

REFERENCES

Dharmendra, 1985, *Leprosy*, Samant and Company, Bombay, vol. 2, p 1223-1227.

Park, J.E.; Park, K., 1989, *Concepts of Health and Disease*, Banarsidas Bhanot, Jabalpur, p 11-44.

WHA, 1991, *Forty-fourth World Health Assembly*, Agenda Item 17.2, WHA 44.9.

WHO, 1991, *Towards Elimination of Leprosy*, Leprosy Control Programme, World Health Organisation, WHO/CTD/LEP/91.1.

PART II

GLOBAL VIEW

2

GLOBAL LEPROSY SITUATION: An Overview

R.S. MISRA

Leprosy is a disease of antiquity. The accurate description of the clinical manifestations of the disease and its treatment are available in one of the oldest Indian Medicinal text, *Susruta Samhita*, 600 B.C. The disease, at one time or the other in the past, was prevalent all over the world, but from most of the European countries it disappeared after 15th century, much before the advent of effective bactericidal drugs against its causative organism. The reasons for it have always been the subject-matter of inquisitiveness to scientists of all hues, viz., medical, social, etc. Even Hansen, the discoverer of the leprosy bacillus confirmed it by his observation in 1888 that the descendants of the Norwegians, who had emigrated from Norway to the USA had no leprosy, opining therefrom that this was largely due to their better social and living conditions. A look at the world map brings to focus one fact very clearly that even today the countries where leprosy is endemic are situated around equatorial belt. It is another added fact that these countries share amongst themselves being underdeveloped or developing in the economic order of today's world.

Quantum of Leprosy Problem

Leprosy being a disease with chronic course and many undeterminable variables, like incubation period, non-availability of laboratory culture medium, objective and precise diagnostic criteria for its earliest incipient stages, was considered for long a static disease, rather to be more true, ever-worsening, in terms of increasing number of patients. Most estimates are made on very inadequate information from limited areas of the regions and on the basis of total registered cases. From these, estimates of prevalence are extrapolated after applying certain arbitrary correction factors.

TABLE 2.1: WHO Estimates for Leprosy

Year	Total Estimate (in million)
1966	10.8
1976	10.6
1982	11.5

Source: Based on WHO, 1991.

Although no estimate has been made in the current decade, it is most likely that the current world leprosy figures will be lower than the 1982 figures because of introduction of multi-drug therapy (MDT) during this decade. The specified duration of treatment regimen has begun a process of deletion of leprosy cases from clinic registers, responsible for the decline in leprosy estimates.

Population at Risk

Approximately 1320 million people live in 28 countries where leprosy is a serious problem, i.e., the registered prevalence is over one case per 1000 persons, and thus may be considered as at significant risk of contracting the disease.

Registered Cases

The information based on registered cases of leprosy gives us much more accurate information with regard to actual quantum of problem at hand than the number of estimated cases. There had been a steady increase in the number of registered cases between 1966 and 1985, with a decline since then, obviously due to implementation of fixed time schedule MDT (Table 2.2).

TABLE 2.2: Registered Cases in the World : Year-wise

Year	Total Registered Cases
1966	2,831,775
1976	3,599,949
1985	5,368,202
1990	3,737,375

Source: Based on WHO, 1991.

The introduction of MDT and its completion over a fixed time schedule has resulted in 30 per cent reduction in registered cases over 1985 figures (Table 2.3).

TABLE 2.3: Distribution of Registered Leprosy Cases, by WHO Region, 1990

WHO Region	Registered Cases	Prevalence per 10000	Percentage of total	New Cases Detected	Case Detection per 10000
Africa	482,669	9.20	12.91	37,335	0.71
Americas	301,704	4.20	8.08	30,543	0.42
South-East Asia	2,693,104	20.50	72.06	488,285	3.72
Europe	7,246	0.10	0.19	87	0.00
Eastern Mediterranean	99,913	2.60	2.67	6,008	0.15
Western Pacific	152,739	1.00	4.09	14,103	0.09

Source: Based on WHO, 1991.

New Case Detection

The relationship between the number of registered cases and the annual number of new cases detected provides (i) useful information on the effectiveness of case-detection activities, and (ii) alertness and viability of the control programme in the region. Though only a proportion of estimated cases are registered for treatment, it reflects in a large measure the leprosy situation in any given region, *vis-a-vis*, other regions.

The number of new cases detected in 1989 was about 5,80,000, indicating a case detection rate of about 1 per 10,000 population. A large majority of these new cases were detected from the South-East Asia region, which contributes the largest share of registered cases in the world. It had shown a dramatic increase between 1966 and 1985 with a steep decline in 1990. A large proportion of the cases and trends towards change for the reduction in prevalence are from India.

In contrast to it, the African region shows a steady decline in the number of registered cases over the past two and half decades. The reasons for it need to be sought for definitively, either in terms of reduced case finding activities or to a true reduction, or to both.

Another hyper-endemic region where there is increase in the number of registered cases comparable to South-East Asia is the

American region. Here a major proportion of this increase is contributed by Brazil.

Leprosy Hyper-endemic Regions of the World

Leprosy in some measure is prevalent all over the world. Though every individual patient anywhere needs immediate medical attention, yet a concerted uniform approach is to be devised in areas where it poses a health problem in terms of numbers due to its antecedent infectious and communicable character. Arbitrarily a prevalence of one case per 1000 population in an area may be considered endemic from the point of view of enforcing a control/eradication programme. Conforming to the above criterion the countries in the world regions mentioned in Tables 2.4 to 2.9 fall in the group.

TABLE 2.4: Population Estimates: Distribution of Registered Cases by WHO Region, 1990

WHO Region	Population (latest official estimate) ('000)	Registered Cases	
		Number	Prevalence rate per 1000
Africa	522,475	482,669	0.92
Americas	724,002	301,704	0.42
Eastern Mediterranean	391,460	99,913	0.26
Europe	845,948	7,246	0.01
South-East Asia	1,310,847	2,693,104	2.05
Western Pacific	1,497,539	152,739	0.10

Source: Based on WHO, 1991.

TABLE 2.5: Prevalence Rate above 1 per 1000 : WHO South-East Asia Region

Countries/Areas	Registered Cases	Prevalence per 10,000
India	2,370,087	27.70
Maldives	388	18.00
Myanmar	134,487	32.30
Nepal	25,361	13.20

Source: Based on WHO, 1991.

TABLE 2.6: Prevalence Rate above 1 per 1000 : WHO African Region

Countries/Areas	Registered Cases	Prevalence per 10,000
Benin	5,655	11.90
Burkina Faso	13,312	14.80
Cameroon	12,302	10.90
Cape Verde	491	12.90
Central African Republic	7,096	24.40
Chad	10,651	18.80
Congo	6,416	32.20
Cote d'Ivoire	24,691	19.30
Gabon	2,491	21.30
Guinea	15,818	23.00
Guinea Bissau	1,179	11.90
Liberia	4,589	18.00
Madagascar	19,210	16.00
Mali	22,121	23.60
Mozambique	24,338	15.50
Nigeria	1,93,715	17.10
Senegal	11,554	15.70
Togo	3,987	11.50

Source: Based on WHO, 1991.

TABLE 2.7: Prevalence Rate above 1 per 1000: WHO Region of the Americas

Countries/Areas	Registered Cases	Prevalence per 10,000
Brazil	239,862	10.00

Source: Based on, WHO, 1991.

TABLE 2.8: Prevalence Rate above 1 per 1000: WHO Eastern Mediterranean Region

Countries/Areas	Registered Cases	Prevalence per 10,000
Sudan	51,716	20.50

Source: Based on WHO, 1991.

TABLE 2.9: Prevalence Rate above 1 per 1000: WHO Western Pacific Region

Countries/Areas	Registered Cases	Prevalence per 10,000
American Samoa	62	16.20
Kiribati	72	10.50
Pacific Islands Trust Territories	707	40.90
Papua New Guinea	6,345	15.80

Source: Based on WHO, 1991.

In terms of total number of registered cases and high prevalence rates, WHO South-East Asian region followed by WHO African region are the worst affected. The total number of registered cases in South-East Asia region is 2,693,104 with a prevalence of 2.05 per 1000 population (Table 2.4). The African region in comparison has second largest number of 482,669 registered cases and overall prevalence of 9.20 per 10,000 population (Table 2.4). Nearly 72 per cent of the registered cases in the world are found in the South-East Asia region.

Amongst the various countries of the world India individually has got around two-thirds of the world population of registered leprosy patients distributed over a vast area in terms of its territory. Along with India other countries in the South-East Asia region with more than 1/1000 prevalence are Maldives, Myanmar and Nepal (Table 2.5).

In the WHO African region Nigeria has the highest number of Registered leprosy cases, i.e., 1,93,715 with a prevalence of 1.7 per 1000 population. Though a number of countries in the region have more than 1/1000 prevalence, yet the total number of registered cases in them are comparatively small (Table 2.6). In the Americas, Brazil has 2,39,862 registered cases with a prevalence of 1/1000 (Table 2.7). In the Eastern Mediterranean region Sudan is the only country with 2.05/1000 prevalence (Table 2.8). In the Western Pacific Papua New Guinea has got the highest number of registered cases, and other countries in the region sharing more than 1/1000 prevalence are, American Samoa, Kiribati and Pacific Islands Trust Territories (Table 2.9).

MDT as Accepted Line of Treatment

MDT was introduced in the leprosy control programme in early eighties. The review of past six to seven years shows that the progress with implementation of MDT has rapidly increased over the period and the percentage of leprosy cases under MDT has shown a marked upward trend. Not only this, more and more leprosy cases are being discharged from treatment after cure with MDT (Table 2.10).

Though the implementation of MDT in various regions of the world had not been uniform, yet this had been of a high order in the most endemic region, i.e., the South-East Asian region. As much as 81.3 per cent of registered cases have been put on MDT in this region. But the implementation of MDT, in other world regions, except Western Pacific has remained below optimum (Table 2.11).

TABLE 2.10: Progress with Implementation of Multidrug Therapy (MDT)

Year	Oct. 1985	Oct. 1986	Oct. 1987	Oct. 1988	Oct. 1989	Oct. 1990	Oct. 1991
Registered cases (000s)	5368	5341	5078	4908	3866	3737	3205
No. of cases on MDT	78752	468222	1318964	1604927	1751903	2080998	2161045
% of total cases on MDT	1.47	8.77	25.97	32.70	45.32	55.69	67.42
No. of cases who completed MDT (cumulative total)	9425	93216	515144	627919	853706	1204825	1411468

Source: Noordeen, 1991.

TABLE 2.11: MDT Coverage by WHO Regions, October 1991

WHO region	No. of Registered Cases*	No. of Cases on MDT	% of registered cases on MDT	No. of cases of completed MDT
Africa (AFR)	361	96635	26.8	127117
Americas (AMR)	336	69463	20.7	28630
Eastern Mediterranean (EMR)	93	34691	37.4	19486
Europe (EUR)	7	2329	33.2	2445
South-East Asia (SEAR)	2276	1851491	81.3	1151391
Western Pacific (WPR)	132	106436	80.7	82399
Total	3205	2161045	67.4	1411468

* in thousands.

Source: Noordeen, 1991.

The MDT has given a new found hope in the treatment of leprosy because of :

(1) The fixed, comparatively short and certain treatment of leprosy with very low relapse rates following completion of therapy; and

(2) Increased self-reporting of leprosy cases at an early stage of

the disease on observing the successful cure of other leprosy patients, with likely reduction in the number and degree of deformities in future.

Disability amongst Leprosy Cases

It is estimated that there are about two to three million individuals in the world who are disabled physically and socially as a result of either past or present affliction with leprosy. A large proportion of these disabled persons will survive the turn of the century, besides addition of a significant proportion of new cases occurring in 1990s and some old patients developing deformities resulting from late diagnosis and insufficient care (Noordeen, 1992).

Thus, even after attainment of abacterial state for a majority of leprosy patients and eliminating leprosy as a public health problem, the problem of disability will persist which will make it difficult to completely eliminate social stigma against leprosy.

Elimination by the Year 2000

The 44th World Health Assembly in May 1991 adopted a resolution on the elimination of leprosy by the year 2000. It defined the elimination as attaining a level of prevalence below one case per 10,000 population. In this context it urged Member States to increase their political commitment for leprosy in order to reach the elimination goal, and requested the Director General of WHO to strengthen technical support to Member States and to continue to mobilise and coordinate resources from Non-governmental Organisations and others in order to achieve the goal (WHA, 1991).

REFERENCES

Noordeen, S.K., 1991, Elimination of Leprosy as a Public Health Problem, *Ind J Lepr*, 63 (3-4), p. 401-409.

Noordeen, S.K., 1992, Elimination of Leprosy as a Public Health Problem, *Lepr Rev*, 63, p. 1-4, editorial.

WHA, 1991, *Forty-fourth World Health Assembly Resolution*, Agenda Item 17.2 WHA 44.9.

WHO, 1991, *Report of the WHO Intercountry Consultative Meeting of Leprosy Programme Managers*, Kathmandu, Nepal, 17-21, December 1990, SEA/Lep/115, 27th March, 1991, Restricted.

WHSQ, 1991, *World Health Statistics Quarterly*, vol 44, no. 1.

3

HIGH-ENDEMIC WORLD REGIONS FOR LEPROSY

R.S. MISRA

In terms of vast population at risk, total number of registered leprosy cases, prevalence rates, detection of new cases and case detection rate, the South-East Asia (SEA) region, African Region and American region are the highly affected regions of the world in descending order. Using the 1990 mid-year population data Table 3.1 illustrates this point.

TABLE 3.1: High-Endemic World Regions for Leprosy

WHO Region	Registered Cases	Prevalence per 1000	% of total	New Case detection	Case detection per 10000
South-East Asia Region	2,693,104	2.50	72.06	488,285	3.72
African Region	482,669	0.92	12.91	37,335	0.71
American Region	301,704	0.42	8.08	30,543	0.42

Source: Based on WHSQ, 1991.

Approximately 1.3 billion people are in high risk population group for leprosy, because they live in areas where leprosy is an important problem, meaning thereby, that the estimated prevalence is over 1 case per 1000 persons in the population.

I. SEA Region

Amongst the various regions of the world, SEA region is the most populous. India, as one of the countries in the region, has the second largest world population as a country following China. There are nine countries included in the region, with four, namely, India, Myanmar, Maldives and Nepal, having a high prevalence rate above 1 per 1000 population (Table 3.2).

TABLE 3.2: Countries in SEA Region with > > 1/1000 Prevalence of Leprosy

Countries	Registered Cases	Prevalence/10000
India	23,70,687	27.70
Maldives	388	18.00
Myanmar	1,34,487	32.30
Nepal	25,361	13.20

Note: Except for India (1990), figure for the rest of the countries are based on 1989 data.

Source: Based on WHSQ, 1991.

India has a high prevalence of paucibacillary (PB) leprosy as compared to multibacillary (MB) (21.3% only) in contrast to Myanmar (previously Burma) (43.89%). Bhutan (57.6%), Sri Lanka (32.2%) and Thailand (66.67%), which have a high Multi-bacillary (MB) case load. Deformities as a sequale of leprosy are reported as very high from Bhutan (actual figures not available), Myanmar (25.78%), Thailand (27%) and Nepal (12%) in the region (Table 3.3).

TABLE 3.3: Child and Deformity Ratio Expressed in Percentage in Various Countries of the Region

Countries	Parameters		
	MB %	Child Rate %	Deformity Rate %
Bhutan	57.6	10.2	very high
India	21.3	16.3	2.7
Indonesia	44	20	10
Maldives	14	1.7	—
Myanmar	43.89	3.87	25.78
Nepal	—	5.57	12
Sri Lanka	32.2	17.7	3
Thailand	66.67	3	27

Source: Based on WHO, 1991.

SITUATIONAL ANALYSIS OF COUNTRIES

I. SEA Region

1. *India*

India has the largest population (approx. 843.93 million) in the region with its vast geographical area and one-third of the total estimated leprosy patients. Due to intensified and effective leprosy eradication programme, the prevalence has fallen from estimated four million in 1981 to three million in 1990. The endemicity of the disease is variable in various parts of the country. There is a vertical National Leprosy Eradication Programme (NLEP) in high-endemic (5+ per 1000 population) districts. There are 196 such districts out of a total of 445 districts in the country.

Annually, about 450,000 new leprosy cases are being detected. Since 1987, a progressive decline in the prevalence of the disease is registered due to number of cases discharged being more than the new cases detected. In the year ending 1990, 2.46 million cases remain on record registers and by March 1991 it had further come down to 2.06 million. Various voluntary agencies are doing yeoman service in collaborating with the NLEP of the Government of India and implementing multi-drug therapy (MDT).

Out of 196 endemic districts, 130 districts have been brought under MDT. It is proposed to bring the remaining 66 endemic districts under MDT by partially integrating the services with Primary Health Care (PHC), through a modified MDT scheme. Under the modified MDT scheme, patients coming to collect drugs and completing the regular MDT will be given monetary compensation.

The leprosy programme is evaluated independently in alternate years, jointly by the World Health Organisation (WHO) and the Government of India.

2. *Myanmar* (previously called *Burma*)

Myanmar has a population of 40 million and comprises 14 States/divisions divided into 314 townships. There is an estimated case-load of 700,000 patients. Currently (June 1990) 120,000 cases are registered. The MB ratio (43.89%) and deformity rate (25.87%) are very high as compared to other countries of the region.

Like India, the programme started as a vertical programme with dapsone therapy in 1955 and attained a 100 per cent coverage by control programme in 1964. In 1978 all disease control programmes, including leprosy, were integrated with PHC services, who undertook the task of distributing dapsone to the patients. Thirty per cent of the vertical personnel were deployed in the PHC services as multipurpose workers.

Six hyperendemic divisions out of 14 were brought under MDT. The MDT was implemented by vertical programme personnel only. In future, it is proposed to expand the MDT coverage in the existing area to achieve a 100 per cent coverage and utilise PHC personnel for expansion of the leprosy activities by training the PHC workers at various levels.

3. *Nepal*

Nepal has an estimated population of 18 million. Leprosy is a formidable public health problem in the country with 25.361 registered cases and a prevalence rate of 13.20 per 10,000 population — MB ratio is considered high, though no figures are available. The country has introduced MDT and so far 52 per cent of registered cases have been brought under it.

The objectives of the national programme are to reduce the prevalence rate from 1.4/1000 to 0.1/1000 population by the year 2000 and provide the MDT coverage to leprosy patients throughout the country by ensuring the adequate supplies of the drugs at district headquarters.

4. *Maldives*

Maldives is the smallest country in the region with a prevalence of eighteen per 10,000 population and 388 registered cases.

The monotherapy was in vogue since 1959, but in 1976 a leprosy control programme was started. Under it, all islands of the Republic except Male, the capital, were surveyed for leprosy, covering 9.7 per cent of total population. MB leprosy is only 14 per cent. Since the introduction of MDT in 1982, leprosy has declined considerably.

A plan of action for zero transmission of disease by 1995 has been drawn up and put into action with early detection and treatment of all new cases. Total leprosy cases coverage for MDT and their monitoring and chemoprephylaxis of the population with single dose rifampicin has been established.

The programme is implemented by PHC mobile team, which visits every island of the country at least four times a year.

5. *Bhutan*

Bhutan has a prevalence of only 2.60 per 10,000 population and 399 registered cases. The MB leprosy is predominant (57.6%). Socio-geographical factors come in the way of effective operations and skin-colour-effects deter some patients from taking clofazimine regularly.

6. *Indonesia*

Indonesia with a prevalence of 6.70 per 10,000 population has the third highest (121,512), registered cases in the region with 44 per cent leprosy and high child ratio.

The MDT is being introduced in a phased manner in collaboration with Netherlands Leprosy Relief Association, WHO and CIBA-Geigy. During the 1990-1994 period, 80 per cent of the registered cases and all new cases are to be put under MDT.

It is expected to reduce the prevalence of the disease to 1/10,000 population by the year 2000.

7. *Sri Lanka*

It has a prevalence of 1.40/10,000 population and 32.2 per cent MB leprosy and a high childhood leprosy (17.7%). The programme funded by International Voluntary Agencies, WHO and the National Ministry suffers from understaffing. The deficiency is being bridged by training the PHC staff and practising doctors, and supplying them with MDT blister packs for free supply to patients. In return they are asked to furnish patient information anonymously.

The programme aims at interrupting the transmission of disease and destigmatising leprosy by increased health education activities, in order to encourage self-reporting.

8. *Thailand*

Thailand, with a prevalence of 3 per 10,000 population, has 16,663 registered cases of leprosy. Under the Leprosy Control Programme started in 1955, a national randomised survey revealed an estimated prevalence of 5/1000 and 140,000 total leprosy cases in the country.

An intensive vertical programme, between 1955-1970 based on intensive case-finding together with domiciliary treatment and follow-up, reduced the prevalence to 1.24/1000 population by the year 1970. Afterwards, under a comprehensive health care system the programme was integrated with PHC set-up with supervision, support and supplementary activities provided by leprosy zonal centres.

MDT operation has been in progress since 1984 covering 92 per cent of registered cases. It has succeeded in impressively bringing down the prevalence to 0.24/1000 in the year 1990. It is proposed to launch a disability prevention and rehabilitation programme in future along with development of biomedical research activities in the field of immunology to further strengthen the programme, with an aim to achieve the goal of eradication of leprosy by the year 2000.

9. *Bangladesh*

It has a prevalence of 1.80 per 10,000 population and a total of 21,191 registered cases of leprosy. Fifty-four per cent leprosy cases have been brought under MDT covering a large size of leprosy population. The problem is being actively addressed to and in the targeted year of 2000 it may be possible to bring down the prevalence to the desired limits.

II. WHO African Region

The WHO African Region with a population of 500 million has 482,669 registered cases, representing 13 per cent of the total leprosy population which is the second highest amongst the world WHO regions with a prevalence of 0.92 per 1000. The leprosy control, started in the 1960s as a vertical programme on monotherapy, is being integrated with PHC and modified to MDT because of the emergence of dapsone resistance. The data on distribution of patients according to age, sex or type of leprosy are very limited.

Nigeria alone accounts for 40 per cent of patients in the region.

The whole region can be divided into the following three sub-regions.

Sub-region I

Comprises 18 countries situated in the north-west and west. It has twice the prevalence rate as that of other sub-regions and a total of abut 320,000 patients. The prevalence of disease, during the past 20 years has considerably declined. It could be attributed to various factors, like, high population increase, decline in the incidence of disease, updating of available data, reduction in detection activities, etc. The programme is being transformed from a vertical specialised system to an integrated one, by making available MDT in general health units.

Sub-region II

Comprises 13 countries in the Central and Eastern regions. It has for long been considered a very high prevalence area. In recent years prevalence has declined sharply to 0.7 per 1000. The programme in the area is mainly vertical. The implementation of MDT had been very slow, except in Ethiopia.

Sub-region III

Comprises 16 countries in the Southern part of the continent. The leprosy has declined considerably in recent years. MDT coverage in the sub-region had been higher than the other two sub-regions.

Countries with More than 1 per 1000 Prevalence in the WHO African Region

Table 3.4 summarises the information with regard to total number of cases, their break-up into PB and MB, if available, prevalence and case detection rate per 10,000 population and percentage of MDT coverage of the population. An outline of the nature of the Control Programme, whether vertical, integrated into other priority special programmes in the country or into PHC or general health care set-up is made. Table 3.4 also indicates the year of introduction of MDT in the country and future planning.

TABLE 3.4: Countries with More than 1 per 1000 Prevalence in the WHO African Region

Country	No. of Cases			Prevalence Rate*	Case-Detection Rate*	MDT Coverrage %	Control Programme Status	Year MDT Introduced
	PB	MB	Total					
1	2	3	4	5	6	7	8	9
1. Cameroon	9085	3217	12302	10.9	0.96	35.3	Completed integrated into the General Health Service.	—
2. Gabon	NA	NA	2491	21.3	1.3	52	—	—
3. Guinea Bissau	618	418 143NK	1179	11.9	2.13	100	Since 1980 combined with TB. Progressively integrated into PHC.	1986
4. Benin	2221	1825	4046	11.9	1.5	30.4	Still vertical. MDT resulted in sharp drop in prevalence.	1987
5. Burkina Faso	11010	2302	13312	14.8	1.65	8	Partly integrated. Specialised personnel at intermediate level.	1990
6. Cape Verde	—	—	491	12.9	1	13	—	—
7. CAR	5707	1389	7096	24.4	1.5	29.4	Combined with TB and Trypanosomiasis.	1986
8. Chad	8926	1725	10651	18.8	0.9	6.3	Partly integrated. Specialized mobile teams for detection activities.	1984

Contd.

TABLE 3.4 *Contd.*

1	2	3	4	5	6	7	8	9
9. Congo	NA	NA	6416	32.2	1	3.8	Partly integrated or still vertical and combined with TB, Trypanosomiasis, Schistosomiasis, Immunization.	1985
10. Cote d'Ivoire	20669	3622	24291	19.3	1.8	9.5	In the process of being integrated.	1983
11. Guinea	1871	376 13571 NK	155818	23.0	1.3	14.0	PHC approach.	1986
12. Mali	17874	4247	22121	23.6	1.7	3.3	Integrated PHC	1987
13. Mozambique	830	731 22777NK	24338	15.5	0.9	6.4	Combined with TB. Partially into General Health Structure.	1984
14. Nigeria	44609	12078 137028NK	193715	17.1	0.5	4.3	Accounts for > 40% cases in the Region. Integrated with PHC.	1985
15. Senegal	7580	3974	11554	15.7	0.7	12.6	Vertical.	1986
16. Togo	2504	1483	3987	11.5	1.3	4.7	Vertical. Plans to expand MDT in whole country by 1995. Integrated into General Health Services.	

* per 10,000 NA = Not available NK = Not known CAR = Central African Republic

Source: Based on WHSQ, 1991.

The disease prevalence is variable in the more than one per 1000 prevalence countries of the region. The case-detection rate is much low and demand more intensive inputs in the area. The MDT coverage, so far, had been poor to make an effective dent in the control of the disease in the region. It has been attributed mainly to the operational aspects of leprosy control in a difficult socio-economic background.

The result of some surveys and programmes in the region have provided useful information. According to them, the leprosy in children below 15 years of age among new cases is 25-40 per cent, while among new cases is about 10 per cent.

To combat the problem of leprosy control in an effective manner within a limited time range, the Inter-regional Conference on Leprosy Control in Africa, held in November 1989 had made important recommendations in the matter.

REFERENCES

WHO, 1991, *Report of the WHO Intercountry Consultative Meeting of Leprosy Programme Managers, Kathmandu, Nepal, 17-21 December, 1990* GEA/LEP/115, Restricted

WHSQ, 1991, Leprosy is the WHO African Region, *World Health Statistics Quarterly:* 44, p.16-22.

4

LEPROSY IN AFRICA

A. COLIN McDOUGALL

The African Region (AFRO) of the World Health Organisation (WHO) comprises virtually all the countries of the continent, with the exception of Egypt, Somalia and the Sudan, which are included in the Eastern Mediterranean Region (EMRO). The overall situation with regard to leprosy control in Africa and the implementation of multiple-drug therapy (MDT) as recommended by WHO in 1982 (WHO, 1982) is characterised by a remarkable variation from one country to another. Some, for instance Malawi and Zambia, have highly developed leprosy control programmes with trained staff and have already treated a high percentage of all known cases, and new cases, with MDT. Such countries have made considerable progress towards the goal of elimination of leprosy as a serious public health problem (WHO, 1991) defined as a prevalence figure of one case per thousand or less, of the population, and a yearly incidence of one new case, or less, per 100,000 of the population. Others, by contrast, have poorly developed control programmes, inadequate staff, and have barely started to implement MDT on a meaningful scale. These remarkable differences may be explained to some extent by the obvious contrasts between north and south, east and west, in such an enormous land mass, including differences in ethnic, cultural, political, religious and socio-economic conditions. But at a medical or technical level, the situation is further complicated by a number of impediments including the absence of a good plan of action, inadequate staff, and problems with drug procurement and distribution.

In an effort to fully discuss these problems and to find solutions, a meeting of particular importance was held in Brazzaville, Congo, Africa, in November 1989 and subsequently reported in a WHO document entitled *Report of the Inter-Regional Conference on Leprosy control in Africa* (WHO, 1989). Its main objectives were to examine progress with regard to leprosy control in Africa, including the implementation of MDT, within the primary health care system, whilst at the same time giving attention to the development of (1) strategies for the wider implementation of MDT under varying (and often difficult) circumstances, and (2) mechanisms to ensure maximum cooperation and effectiveness between government and non-government organisations.

The Extent and Distribution of Leprosy in Africa

The total population of the AFRO region is about 500 million and at the end of 1988, 483,435 leprosy patients were registered for treatment, giving a prevalence rate of about 1 case per 1000 and a detection rate of about 8 per 100,000 inhabitants (WHO, 1989). About 40 per cent of all cases are in Nigeria. Prevalence rates above 1 per 1000 (i.e., above 10 per 10,000) for Africa are given in Table 2.5 in Chapter 2 on Global Leprosy Situation.

In a recent WHO publication Daumerie has proposed a classification of the leprosy-endemic countries of Africa, according to endemicity level and MDT coverage (Daumerie, 1991). *Level I* has low endemicity/high MDT coverage and includes Algeria, Botswana, Burundi, Mauritius, Namibia, South Africa and Zimbabwe. *Level IIA* has medium endemicity/MDT coverage > 75 per cent and includes Angola, Comoros, Equatorial Guinea, Gambia, Malawi, United Republic of Tanzania and Zambia. *Level IIB* has medium endemicity/MDT coverage ≤75 per cent and includes Ethiopia, Ghana, Kenya, Lesotho, Mauritania, Niger, Reunion, Rwanda, Seychelles, Sierra Leone, Swaziland, Uganda and Zaire. *Level IIIA* has high endemicity/MDT coverage > 33 per cent and includes Cameroon, Gabon, Guinea Bissau and Madagascar. Finally, *Level IIIB* has high endemicity/MDT coverage ≤ 33 per cent and includes Benin, Burkina Faso, Cape Verde, Central African Republic, Chad, Congo, Côte d'Ivoire, Guinea, Mali, Mozambique, Nigeria, Senegal and Togo. Overall, less than 20 per cent of all known leprosy cases in Africa are being treated with MDT and only 103,000 have so far completed their regimens of treatment. For reasons which will be discussed below, it is clear that coverage varies markedly from one country to another and that some have made considerable progress.

However, the overall picture is disappointing — of the 21 countries worldwide with MDT coverage below 25 per cent, no fewer than 14 are in the AFRO region.

Constraints to Leprosy Control and MDT Implementation

The total number of factors militating against progress in Africa is large, but the following are amongst the most important —

(1) lack of political will and support at the top;
(2) the absence of a good plan of action;
(3) wrong setting of priorities, both with regard to leprosy in comparison with other demands on the health services, but also with regard to various activities within the leprosy programme;
(4) disagreement on technical aspects, including drug combinations and periods of treatment;
(5) lack of coordination between governments and non-government agencies; and
(6) a range of administrative, operational and managerial problems, all of outstanding importance in leprosy-endemic countries which experience difficulties in making progress.

In many circumstances, one must also add to the above list — problems with transport, laboratory services, facilities for the referral or complicated cases and the procurement and distribution of drugs for MDT. Based on prevalence rates, priority for support in solving these problems should go to — Angola, Côte d'Ivoire, Madagascar, Mali, Mozambique, Uganda and Zaire.

Prospects for Improved Leprosy Control in Africa

To many outside observers, the current achievement of many African countries in the development of effective leprosy control programmes and the implementation of MDT is both disappointing and disconcerting. The basic methodology of leprosy control has been well known (and published) for at least 20 years and it has been greatly strengthened by concept and implementation of MDT, as described by WHO in 1982 (WHO, 1982). Furthermore, a number of non-government, international and voluntary organisations, notably those in the International Federation of Anti-Leprosy Associations (ILEP), 234 Blythe Road, London W14 OHJ, England, are available for technical input and financial support, particularly for programmes able or willing to implement MDT according to WHO recommendations, whilst at the same time taking steps for the prevention of disability due to nerve damage. Nevertheless, it has to be acknowledged that in some countries socio-economic and political conditions still represent a formidable barrier to progress, which cannot be overcome by purely medical or technical means. Elsewhere, it remains true to say that much could be done to improve the situation, and to define the totals of patients who (1) are in need of MDT, (2) have completed a satisfactory course of MDT, but are under surveillance, and (3) do not need MDT or surveillance, but who need continuing care (perhaps on a long-term basis) because of disabilities (WHO, 1988). Cases which do not fall into any of these categories do not need to be kept on any form of list or register, and can be released. Indeed, the process of sifting or 'cleaning' the registers of all recorded 'cases', prior to the implementation of MDT, has, in all parts of the world where leprosy is endemic, resulted in highly significant reductions in total prevalence figures, before a single capsule or tablet of MDT is given. A further issue of importance with regard to making progress, centres on the advisability of a special (vertical) programme, as opposed to an integrated (horizontal) approach, using the primary health care (PHC) system, with input at district level. The general impression at the time of writing is that where a vertical service is already established and working well, it should be allowed to continue until the disease is at a low level of prevalence and incidence, before handing over to a horizontal countries, including India. For certain leprosy-endemic countries in Africa, including many of those shown in *Level IIIB* above, it has been suggested (Nebout, 1991) that the only really effective approach is to use mobile and specialised teams, whose work would include treating all known cases regularly and for long enough, whilst actively finding and treating new cases.

Leprosy Control and HIV/AIDS in Africa

Despite the appalling, and worsening situation with regard to the number of HIV-positive people in Africa (WHO, 1987), together with those suffering, or already dying from the AIDS syndrome, and the all too obvious association between HIV/AIDS and TB, (Chum, et al, n.d.; Rees, 1988) significant clinical and/or epidemiological associations with leprosy have not yet been reported. Despite a few publications in which coincident HIV infection and leprosy has been described, there is no clear evidence, at the time of writing, that the vast pool of HIV infection in Africa is adversely affecting the clinical course of leprosy in those already infected, the chances of infection, or response to treatment. Whether this is due to some (fortunate) immunological characteristic of leprosy, by which HIV infection does not seriously affect cell-mediated immunity or to the long-drawn-out clinical course of leprosy in most instances, is as yet unclear and will only be revealed by careful monitoring of the clinical and epidemiological situations for many years to come.

Disability, Deformity, Rehabilitation, Social Aspects

The considerable attention given above to control programme methodology and MDT should not detract from the paramount importance of ensuring that all possible is done to prevent disability in leprosy patients, or, at the very least, to minimise deterioration in established disability (Watson, 1986). It has also to be acknowledged that once the 'wave' of MDT has passed (hopefully, in most parts of the world by the year 2000), many leprosy-endemic countries will be left with large number of patients who have completed satisfactory courses of chemotherapy, but who are disabled or deformed and in need of skilled services. It is not too early to plan ahead for the care of these patients in an effective manner, making the greatest possible use of community-based rehabilitation (Helander, et al, 1980) and doing everything possible to avoid their management in leprosy institutions or colonies.

Conclusions

Dr. S.K. Noordeen, Chief, Leprosy Unit, WHO, recently commented:

> There is no doubt that MDT has brought about a major change in our technology for leprosy control. It has also resulted in a new outlook towards the disease, and raised hopes among patients, health workers and programme managers alike. Where the im-

plementation of MDT is vigorous and sustained, the results are extremely gratifying. Problems both technical and operational need to be constantly reviewed and solutions found. The opportunities to markedly reduce leprosy in the next decade are immense. It remains to be seen whether or not we make use of them, and whether or not leprosy will ultimately be eliminated as a health problem as part of the overall goal of *Health for All by the Year 2000* (Noordeen, 1987).

It is now 1992. The operational 'technologies' for establishing and running an effective leprosy control programme, implementing MDT and preventing disability are all well described. Are we doing enough to help the countries of Africa to use these resources towards the elimination of this ancient disease from their continent?

REFERENCES

Chum, H.J.; Nyangulu, D.S.; Salomao, A.; Gninafon, M.; Enarson, D.A, n.d., *Tuberculosis in the 1990's: Tuberculosis and HIV Infection in Africa*, submitted for publication. (Enquiries to Professor D.A. Enarson, International Union Against Tuberculosis and Lung Disease, 68 Boulevard Saint-Michel, 75006, Paris, France.)

Daumerie, D., 1991, Progress in Leprosy Control through Multidrug Therapy, *World Health Statistics*, 44(1), 1991, WHO, Geneva, Switzerland.

Helander, E.; Mendis, P.; Nelson, G., 1980, *Training Disabled People in the Community*, WHO, Geneva, Switzerland.

Nebout, M., 1991, Renforcement de la lutte contre la lèpre par une polychimiotherapie précoce et systematique. *Acta Leprologica*, 7(4), p. 351-57.

Noordeen, S.K., 1987, *Global Rev: v of MDT Implementation*, Paper presented to WHO/SEARO Intercountry Seminar on Implementation and Evaluation of Multidrug Therapy in Leprosy Control Programmes through Primary Health Care, SEARO, New Delhi, 7-11 December, 1987.

Rees, R.J., 1988, Tuberculosis and Leprosy, *British Medical Bulletin*, 44(3), July 1988, published for the British Council by Churchill Livingstone, Edinburgh, London, Melbourne and New York.

WHO, 1982, *Chemotherapy of Leprosy for Control Programmes*, Technical Report Series, No. 675.

WHO, 1987, *Inter-relation of Tropical Diseases and HIV Infection*; Report of an Informal Consultation held at the Kenya Medical Research Institute (Kemri), Nairobi, Kenya, 1-4 December 1987, TDR/GPA/TD-HIV/87.3, UNDP/World Bank/WHO Special Programme for Research and Training in Tropical Diseases (TDR), Geneva, Switzerland.

WHO, 1988, *WHO Expert Committee on Leprosy, Sixth Report*, Technical Report Series 768. 1988, WHO, Geneva, Switzerland.

WHO, 1989, *Report of the Inter-Regional Conference on Leprosy Control in Africa*, Brazzaville, 6-10 November, 1989, WHO/CDS/LEP/89.1, WHO, Geneva, Switzerland.

WHO, 1991, *Towards the Elimination of Leprosy*, Leprosy Control Programme, WHO, Geneva, Switzerland, WHO/CTD/LEP/91.1.

Watson, J., 1986, *Preventing Disability in Leprosy Patients*, The Leprosy Mission International, TALMILEP, 80 Windmill Road, Brentford, Middlesex TW8 OQH, England.

5

LEPROSY IN BRAZIL

5.1 BRAZIL: THE COUNTRY, ITS PEOPLE AND THE HANSEN'S DISEASE CONTROL PROGRAMME

MARIA DA GRAÇA CUNHA, GERSON OLIVEIRA PENNA
and GERSON FERNANDO MENDES

5.1.1 Country Profile

Brazil, the fifth largest nation in the world and the third largest in the Americas, covers 8,511,996 km^2. With most of its territory between the equator and the tropic of Capricorn, its climate is predominately tropical and subtropical, with a small temperate zone in the south. Brazil has a small coastal plain and two major river plains, the Amazon and Parana river basins; the rest of the country is a plateau averaging about 1000m of altitude. The big east-west dimension encompasses four time-zones. The country has borders with all the South American countries except two, Chile and Ecuador.

Brazil is divided in five regions — North, Northeast, Southeast, South and the Centre West — comprising 26 States and the Federal District. Portuguese is the official language, Roman Catholicism the predominant religion and the currency is the Cruzeiro, currently valued at US$1 = Cr$2,900 (May 29, 1992) and losing value at an average rate of 20 per cent each month. In 1990 the mean annual income per capita was US$2,169.[1] The illiteracy rate is 26 per cent and the population between 1970 and 1980 grew by 2.48 per cent.[2]

In spite of being the eighth largest economy in the world, Brazil is still classified as a developing country.

5.1.2 Health Situation

Brazilian health indicators are compatible with the country's stage of development. They have shown some improvement over the past decades, reflecting the progress in health conditions.

	1940	1985-90[3]
Birth rate	...	28.58/1,000
Death rate	...	8.36/1,000
Fertility rate	6.16%	3.46%
Life expectancy at birth	42.74 years	60.08 yrs
Infant mortality 0-12 months	144.73/1,000	87.88/1,000

In 1986, there were 30,872 health establishments — 18,790 public and 12,082 private — including health posts and centres, small general clinics, emergency rooms, district and other hospitals. There were 489,626 beds (1 for each 283 inhabitants) — 106,794 in public facilities and 382,832 in private ones — and one physician for every 1,350 Brazilians.

Estimates show that approximately one-third of the Brazilian population have no regular access to health services. Almost 40 million people have some degree of malnutrition; diarrhoeal diseases affect millions of children and are responsible for 40 per cent of the infant mortality.

As a result of such regional disparities, Brazil has, on one hand, a share of diseases typical of underdeveloped countries such as infectious and parasitic diseases (tuberculosis, Hansen's disease, amoebiasis, malaria, schistosomiasis, etc.) and, on the other, conditions typical of countries with a better quality of life and a higher life expectancy at birth (cancer, circulatory diseases, traffic and other accidents, etc.).

5.1.3 Hansen's Disease Situation in Brazil

5.1.3.1 *Hansen's Disease: An Overview*

The first Hansen's disease cases in Brazil were notified in 1600 in Rio de Janeiro. Other disease focii were identified in Bahia and Para around the same time.

Control activities were started two centuries later, limited to the building of leprosaria and to some precarious assistance to the patients.

Between 1912 and 1920, Hansen's disease was recognised as a public health problem. The sanitary authorities at that time created the Inspectorship for the Prophylaxis of Leprosy and Venereal Diseases. Among control activities, priority was given to the building of leprosaria for the compulsory admission of patients in all endemic States, leprosy census and treatment with chaulmoogra oil.

In 1935, control of the disease took a new direction, with the extension of care to the patients' family members. In 1941, the National Leprosy Service was created.

Measures adopted in Brazil to face the problem were not different from those taken in the rest of the world at that time — compulsory internment, treatment with chaulmoogra, and later with dapsone and rifampicin.

Vertically organised activities and mandatory isolation were not able to control the endemicity, and contributed to increase the fear and the stigma associated with the disease. By the end of the 1960s, mandatory admission was abolished and the National Campaign against Leprosy was dismantled. It was substituted by the National Division of Sanitary Dermatology, based on the recommendation that hierarchic horizontalisation of control actions was fundamental to creating an impact on the endemicity. This point marks the beginning of Hansen's disease control activities' insertion into primary health care (PHC).

In 1982, the Instituto de Dermatologia Tropical "*Alfredo da Matta*" and the Hospital Estadual do Curupaiti (Rio de Janeiro) began to use multiple-drug therapy (MDT) (WHO) in selected patients. Based on this experience, the Ministry of Health started its own National MDT Project in 1986, initially in selected areas. In August 1991, MDT became the only official leprosy therapeutic regimen in the country.

5.1.3.2 *Epidemiological Situation, 1990*

I. Prevalence and Distribution of Hansen's Disease in Brazil: At the end of 1990, there were 278,692 registered cases of Hansen's disease in Brazil — the highest number ever observed. This corresponds to a prevalence rate of 1.85 cases per thousand population, falling into the "high" bracket according to the World Health Organisation criteria.[4] Brazil has approximately 87 per cent of all the Hansen's disease patients in the Americas, and the third largest number of patients in the world.

Among the five regions, four have a high prevalence (North, Centre West, Southeast and South with 4.44, 3.85, 1.74 and 1.23 cases per thousand population respectively). The Northeast has a medium prevalence of 0.92/1,000 population.

Among the Brazilian States, only seven (Rio Grande do Norte, Paraiba, Alagoas, Bahia, Sergipe, Santa Catarina and Rio Grande do Sul) have a medium prevalence rate; in the other twenty States, the prevalence is high. Based on this data, we can state that 76.87 per cent of the Brazilian population, or 115,601,700 people, live in areas with a high prevalence of Hansen's disease.

Of the 278,692 registered cases in 1990, 51.99 per cent (144,885) are lepromatous and borderline, 24.91 per cent (69,418) are tuberculoid, 22.02 per cent (61,378) indeterminate and 0.87 per cent (2,423) are unclassified.

The Northeastern and Southern regions are particularly interesting. The first has the highest proportion of tuberculoid forms (34.48%) and the smallest of lepromatous and borderline ones (41.59%). The second has the highest proportion of lepromatous and borderline forms (61.28%) and the smallest of tuberculoid ones (18.08%). Along with others, these figures point to the possibility of the expansion of endemicity and stabilisation, respectively, in the regions.

In spite of the high detection rate registered in 1990, the number of registered cases increased by only 4.54 per cent in relation to the previous year (266,578). This may be related to the "clearing" of central files, as well as to the increase in the number of discharges as cured (Table 5.1.1).

TABLE 5.1.1: Evolution of Inclusion of HD Cases on MDT/WHO: Brazil, 1985-1991

Years	Total number HD Cases	Patients on MDT No.	%	%Increase from the previous year	%Regularity on MDT
1985	222,797	1,329	0.6	—	—
1986	234,560	5,088	2.2	282,84	—
1987	239,328	9,551	4.0	87,71	94.9
1988	256,979	20,812	8.1	117,90	94.5
1989	245,005	32,330	12.5	55,34	96.8
1990	278,662	50,147	18.0	55,10	86.0
1991	216,034 *	72,034 **	33.59 *	44,70	—

Source: State Health Departments.

* Estimated

** Non cumulative date (excluding discharges as cured and other discharges from active register)

II. **New Cases:** Fig. 5.1.1 shows the evolution of detection rates in the country in the last twenty years.

In 1990, 28,482 new cases of Hansen's disease were registered, corresponding to a detection rate of 18.94/100,000 population. According to the WHO criteria, Brazil is a high detection country ($\geq$ 10/100,000 per year). These were the largest number and highest rate ever observed in Brazil. In relation to 1989, there was a 2.3 per cent increase in detection (27,837 new cases in 1989).

Detection rates by regions decreased progressively from the North, Centre West, Northeast, Southeast to the South, with 49.68, 49.19, 15.67, 13.62 and 6.95 per 100,000 population respectively.

According to the clinical form, of the 28,482 new Hansen's disease cases detected in 1990, 41.64 per cent (11,861) were lepromatous and borderline, 29.41 per cent (8,377) tuberculoid, 27.26 per cent (7,763) indeterminate and 1.69 per cent (481) were not classified. These numbers suggest both a late diagnosis and the expansion of the endemicity.

10.41 per cent of the 28,482 new cases in 1990 were children under 15 years of age, a figure considered high by the WHO whose classification begins at 8 per cent. The North and Northeast and the Centre West, which have respectively the highest prevalence rate and the highest increase trends, also show the highest proportion of children under 15 years of age among new cases (17.36%, 14.32% and 7.99% respectively).

5.1.4 Hansen's Disease Control Programme

MDT was adopted in January 1990 as Brazil's official and preferential therapeutic regimen for Hansen's disease and, as previously mentioned, in August 1991 it became the country's only therapeutic regimen.

5.1.5 Evolution of MDT

At the end of 1990, there were 42,282 cases of Hansen's disease on MDT, corresponding to 17.3 per cent of the total number of registered cases.

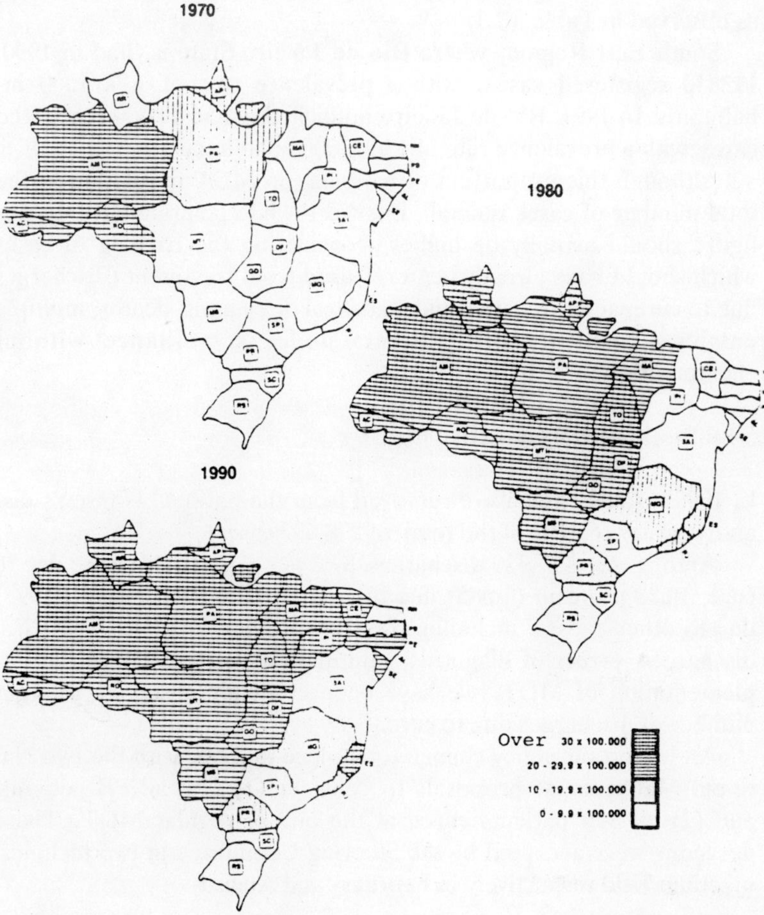

FIG. 5.1.1: Evolution of HD detection Rates : Brazil, 1970-1990

Source: State Health Departments
Ministry of Health/National Health Foundation/National Sanitary Dermatology Management

Brazil finished the year of 1990 with 278,692 leprosy patients registered and with a prevalence rate of 1,85/1000 inhabitants. Until the end of the referred year, 50,147 leprosy patients were included in MDT regimens, representing 18.00 per cent of the registered cases, as observed in Table 5.1.1.

South East Region, where Rio de Janeiro State is, had in 1990, 113840 registered cases, with a prevalence rate of 1,74/1000 inhabitants. In 1991, Rio de Janeiro municipality had 12,404 registered cases, with a prevalence rate of 1,99/1000 inhabitants.

Although this proportion of patients on MDT in relation to the total number of cases is small, it is worthwhile pointing out that this figure should actually be higher, considering the backlog of cases which should have already been released from treatment (discharges due to cure, administrative and statistical discharges, deaths, multiple entries, besides those patients under surveillance without chemotherapy).

5.1.6 **Discharges from Active Register**

In 1990, 17,330 cases were removed from the national Hansen's disease register (6.22% of the total of 278,692 cases).

Among these 17,330 discharges, 37.2 per cent (6,447) were due to cure, 10.88 per cent (1,885) due to death and 51.92 per cent (8,998) due to other causes, including transfer to other countries, statistical discharges, errors of diagnosis, multiple entries, etc. Since the implementation of MDT, we have been gradually observing a larger number of discharges due to cure.

An important policy change took place in 1991, with the two National Management proposals to consider (1) first all PB patients, and (2) all MB patients cured at the end of regular MDT. These decisions were accepted by the Steering Committee in two technical meetings held respectively in February and August.

5.1.7 **Perspectives for Disease Control, 1990-94**

The Brazilian Five-Year Plan for the control of Hansen's disease represents the second part of a work proposal launched in 1986.

In the first stage (1986-89), we worked on the foundation of a control programme (assessment of the true dimension of the problem, development of an information system able to give subsidies for decision-making).

The second stage is based on epidemiological stratification, first of the whole country, later of the States and then of the municipalities, utilising the epidemiological criteria of prevalence, incidence and time trends of the disease at each level, adequated to the local operational capacity to achieve the targets.

Our "Emergency Plan" comprises five following activities:

(1) to diagnose all expected cases;
(2) to start all new cases on MDT;
(3) to give MDT to all eligible old MB cases;
(4) to give BCG to all household contacts of MB patients in the last five years; and
(5) to know the real prevalence, updating all files.

These five activities have different time schedules and quantitative targets for the three different priority groups.

Activities 2 and 3 are already officially implemented, with the adoption of the regimen as the country's only official one. This, as we have said, is an ongoing process.

From the plan's daily execution, during the past two years, two activities have emerged as priorities, recognised by the National Management and debated at the National Training Course for HD Managers which took place in early October 1991. This is the "clearing of files" which will bring about a decrease in prevalence in a short period of time, and the acceleration of MDT implementation, according to the aforementioned recommendations.

In our opinion, prevalence alone may not be an adequate indicator in all situations, and at least two other indicators might be considered when looking at the Hansen's disease problem, namely incidence and behaviour. We would also like to quote Dr. Noordeen in saying that "the problem is far more serious than what is represented by the numbers alone, particularly in terms of the intense human suffering involved resulting from the physical deformities and the related social problems".

NOTES

1. BID (Banco Interamericano de Desenvolvimento), *Folha de Sao Paulo*, October 1991.

2. Ministry for Health, Brasilia.
3. This data expresses national averages; regional statistics show large variations, reflecting each region's different degree of development.
4. i.e., 1-10 cases of Hansen's disease per 1,000 population.

BACKGROUND REFERENCES

Anon, 1991, *Activities report, 1990: Hansen's Disease : An Endemy in the Ascendent*, Brazilian Ministry for Health, National Health Foundation, Brasilia, 1991

Anon, 1991, *Brazilian Report*, Conference of Hansen's Disease Control in the Americas, Brazilian Ministry for Health, National Health Foundation, National Epidemiology Centre, National Sanitary Dermatology Technical Management, Mexico City, October 1991

Anon, 1991, *Plano de Emergencia Nacional Consolidado*, 1991-94, Brazilian Ministry for Health, National Health Foundation, National Epidemiology Centre, National Sanitary Dermatology Technical Management, Brasilia DF

Anon, 1992, *Meeting between Brazil's Ministry of Health/National Sanitary Dermatology Technical Management and Non Governmental Organisations Working together with the Brazilian Hansen's Disease Control Programme*, Brazilian Ministry for Health, National Health Foundation, National Epidemiology Centre, National Sanitary Dermatology Technical Management, Brasilia, March 9-10,1992

5.2 LEPROSY CONTROL IN AMAZONAS STATE: MDT and Early Detection

MARIA DA GRAÇA CUNHA and MARIA DA FATIMA MAROJA

5.2.1 State Profile

The State Amazonas covers 1,564,445 km^2 in the north of Brazil. It is the largest State in the Amazon basin and, occupying 18.38 per cent of Brazil's territory, is the largest in the Federation. With 2,443,313 (1990) people its population density is a low 1.55/km^2. Transport within the State and between it and others is principally fluvial, although there is a fairly comprehensive aerial service covering the bigger towns. In the dry season its capital, Manaus, is linked with several towns and two other State capitals by roads.

There are 70 municipalities widely scattered along the Amazon and its tributaries. The rural populations of these towns are to be found along the river banks and are typically dedicated to extractivism (rubber, Brazil nuts), agriculture (subsistence and cash crops) and fishing. The equator runs through the northern portion of the State. It is hot (average temperature is 26°C) and humid (average annual rainfall 2,500 mm).

Until 20 years ago, State's economy was based principally on extractivism — that of rubber. The establishment of an industrial park and a duty free port in the State's capital, Manaus, at that time commenced a shift in the population's main source of income. By 1990,50 per cent of the Amazonas population was living in Manaus. Even with the industrial boom and the growth of the service sector, the migratory rush (in the 1970s the capital's population growth rate was 7.35 per cent per annum) has saturated labour needs. The workforce's resultant low incomes have favoured the growth of slums around the city.

5.2.2 Health Situation

Although Brazil is classified as "developing" country, the Amazonian Region (the States of Acre, Amapa, Amazonas, Para, Randônia and

Roraima in the country's north) has its share of the diseases typical of underdeveloped countries — parasitoses and infections including tuberculosis, leprosy, amoebiasis, malaria, hepatitis, cholera and leishmaniasis.

Amazonas life expectancy at birth is 62.4 years, and infant mortality was measured at 87.8 per cent in 1987.

There are 220 health centres and rural health posts in the State's health services — 68 in Manaus and 152 in the interior.

5.2.3 **Leprosy Situation**

5.2.3.1 *Past*

In the past, the leprosy control programme was a passive one. Few health centres were involved in leprosy control. With late diagnosis, irregular treatment and the difficulties in tracing contacts, a sample of 35 per cent of all patients diagnosed in 1979 showed that 46 per cent of new cases presented with disabilities. Disabilities were present in only 4.7 per cent of 1991s new cases; 100 per cent were evaluated.

In 1979, leprosy control entered a new phase. The leprosarium built in the 1940s was closed down and a small dispensary for leprosy outpatients, *Alfredo da Matta*, was transformed into the Centre for Dermatology and assumed responsibility for leprosy in the State.

5.2.3.2 *Present*

In 1988 the Centre for Dermatology became the Instituto de dermatologia Tropical *Alfredo da Matta*. The management of the leprosy control programme is the responsibility of its staff and the programme is administratively linked with the Amazonas State Government. 76.8 per cent of programme resources are supplied by the Brazilian Government, 17.6 per cent by the German Leprosy Relief Association (DAHW) and 5.6 per cent by the Catholic Church (figures refer to the period 1980-1991). WHO has been supporting research of therapeutic regimens. There are currently two multicentre field trials being carried out in *Alfredo da Matta* — (1) Fixed duration combined chemotherapy in MB leprosy (commenced in 1987), and (2) Field trial of ofloxacin-containing combined drug regimens in MB and PB leprosy (1992).

Training of programme personnel has been carried out regularly in Manaus and in the interior over the past 8 years, with regular 5-10 day courses on general aspects of the disease and multi-drug therapy. 1,966 health workers were trained by *Alfredo da Matta* staff from 1986 to 1991 (374 health professionals and 1,592 paramedics/rural health agents). The majority of the trained staff work in Amazonas, although many people from other States and countries attend professional courses. Twelve Manaus health centres and clinics participate in the MDT programme. A further 13 health centres do skin examinations and refer suspected cases on to *Alfredo da Matta*.

In the most distant parts of the interior, leprosy control has been attempted with three floating general purpose health centres. These boats give partial health cover to the riverine population twice yearly.

On December 31, 1991, the total case load for the State was 16,528, giving a prevalence of 6.7 cases per thousand Amazonians (compared with 1.8 per cent for Brazil as a whole). In the same year, 1,682 new cases were diagnosed, representing a detection coefficient of 69.0 per 100,000 per year. 47.8 per cent of these were multibacillary and 52.5 per cent paucibacillary. Twenty-five per cent of new cases were under 15 years of age, demonstrating the severity of the State's leprosy situation.

As for the mode of detection, 91.6 per cent of the new cases presented spontaneously, reflecting the depth of the educational work carried out among the population in the last ten years. 94.8 per cent of the new cases were put onto MDT and 5.2 per cent onto other schemes.

5.2.4 MDT Implementation

MDT in Amazonas was started in 1982 at the then Centre for Dermatology *Alfredo da Matta*. By December 1991, a total of 20,217 patients were on or had completed MDT. Of these, 10,743 are still on MDT representing 65 per cent of the State's registered patients.

5.2.4.1 *Difficulties in MDT Implementation and Attempted Solutions*

Most of the municipalities in Amazonas are, territorially, very large, and one of the main difficulties encountered is the time a patient needs to spend to come from a rural zone to a centre for monthly supervised treatment. Over the past three years, rural health agents in a few municipalities have been trained in MDT supervision, and in some interior communities patients need only make the long trip to the town health centres for diagnosis, annual review, treatment of reaction and release from treatment (RFT). Because of the immense distances and the poverty of transport in the interior of Amazonas, it is only through such rural extensions that full MDT implementation will be achieved.

In Manaus, the main difficulty is the low compliance among working patients. As a strategy *Alfredo da Matta* has been opening in the evenings (5 to 8 PM) three times a week since 1989 to facilitate treatment of patients on MDT. Doctors, social workers and nursing auxiliaries from 68 factories have been trained in the diagnosis and treatment of leprosy, and in 21 factories patients are receiving supervised MDT in the workplace.

The country's worsening economic situation — the GDP declined by more than six per cent in the new government's first twelve months — has accentuated another difficulty in the implementation of MDT. Many patients in the capital have become irregular in the taking of their monthly doses because of their inability to pay the bus fares. In these cases, we attempt to transfer their treatment to a clinic nearer their home. As many patients prefer to do their treatment in the centre of reference, they can receive transport passes through the Institute's social services department.

5.2.5 Future Perspectives

A study covering the period 1981-1991 has shown the stabilisation of the incidence of leprosy over the past five years. An intensification of the active search for new cases is being carried out in the slum areas (*favelas*) around Manaus and in the interior towns and rural areas seeking to establish whether this conclusion is in fact epidemiologically sound or merely an operational phenomenon.

The difficulties faced in the implementation of MDT in Amazonas, especially in the rural areas where great distances separate patients from the municipal treatment centres and in the urban area of Manaus, would be overcome with the adoption of therapeutic regimes of shorter duration currently under trial in various research centres.

PART III

INDIAN SCENARIO

6

LEPROSY ERADICATION IN INDIA: Evolution and Progress

R.S. MISRA

India has the largest number of leprosy cases compared to any other country in the world. The first reliable information and estimates about the quantum of the disease were made by leprosy surveys conducted during nineteen twenties and thirties by the British Empire Leprosy Relief Association (predecessor of the present Hind Kusht Nivaran Sangh or the Indian Leprosy Association). These surveys estimated the number of cases during the period at approximately one million. Amongst all the WHO regions, the South East Asian Region and amongst all the countries in the world with high endemicity for leprosy, India has the highest percentage of registered cases to the estimated total leprosy population respectively (WHSQ, 1991). Total registered cases rose steadily from 1951 (1.4 million) up to 1981 (3.9 million) and these began falling due to intensive implementation of multi-drug therapy (MDT) in hyperendemic districts (above 5/1000 prevalence) to 2.4 million in 1990 against an estimated 2.8 to 3 million estimated leprosy cases in 1991 (Figs. 6.1 and 6.2).

The disease is not evenly distributed in different States of the country. There are areas of high prevalence (5 or more per thousand). Andhra Pradesh, Tamil Nadu, Orissa and West Bengal have prevalence of more than 10/000. The areas of moderate prevalence (1 to 5 per thousand) are in the Central and Western parts of India of the Himalayan foot-hills and the areas of low prevalence (below one per thousand) are found mostly in the North-Western parts of the country.

A rough estimate of cases of leprosy in the various States in India, arranged according to degree of endemicity and the estimated average prevalence rates of the disease, is given in Table 6.1.

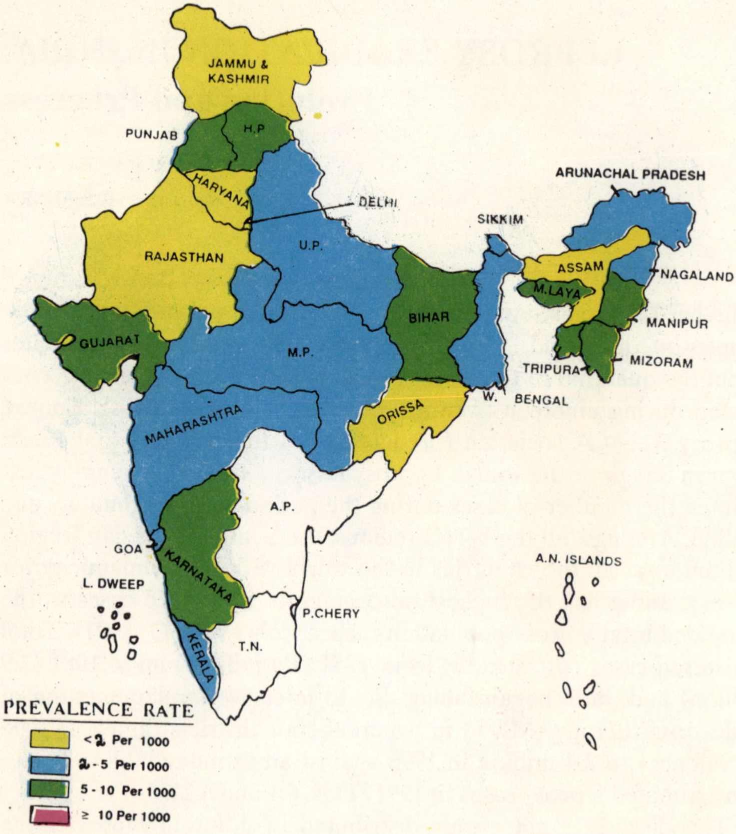

FIG. 6.1: India: Statewise Prevalence of Leprosy, December 31, 1981

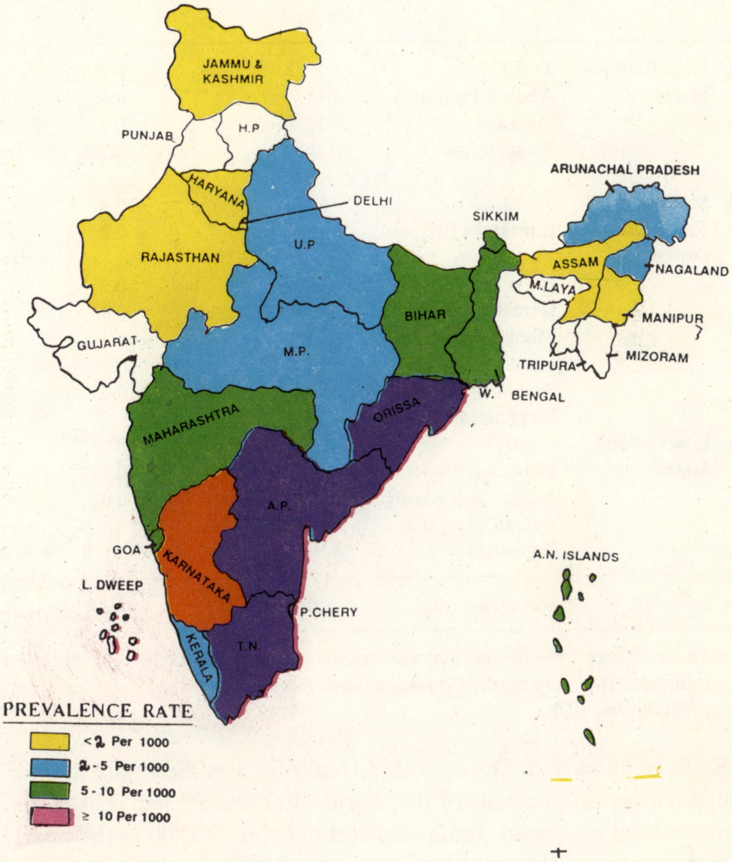

FIG. 6.2: India: Statewise Prevalence of Leprosy as at 1991

TABLE 6.1: Approximate State-wise Distribution of Leprosy in India

Degree of Endemicity	State	Estimated average prevalence rate per thousand	Estimated number of cases in millions
I. High Endemic States	Tamil Nadu	20.0	0.7
	Andhra Pradésh	15.0	0.6
	Orissa	12.0	0.2
	West Bengal	10.00	0.35
II. Moderate Endemic States	Maharashtra	7.5	0.3
	Karnataka (Mysore)	6.5	0.2
	Bihar	6.5	0.3
	Kerala	4.0	0.08
	Madhya Pradesh	3.0	0.1
	Uttar Pradesh	2.5	0.2
	Assam Meghalaya	2.0	0.05
III. Low Endemic States	Gujarat	1.7	0.05
	Himachal Pradesh	1.5	0.05
	Jammu & Kashmir	1.0	0.02
	Punjab, Haryana Rajasthan	0.5	0.3
I+II+III	India (as a whole)	0.50	3.20

* These figures indicate the average prevalence rates for each state; within a state itself there are marked variations in different parts.

Source: Dharendra, 1978.

Eight of India's 26 States with a total of 2.3 million patients, account for over 60 per cent of the world total and 98 per cent of the country's total case-load. India also accounts for 470,000 of the nearly 600,000 new cases currently detected annually throughout the world.

Of the 450 districts in the country, 201 are hyperendemic for leprosy with prevalence of five and more per thousand of population, accounting for more than 50 per cent of the total Indian population at a greater risk for contracting the disease. Child population below 14 years of age accounts for 15 to 20 per cent of the leprosy cases. Around 10-15 per cent of leprosy cases on treatment and released from treatment surveillance suffer with deformities of varying degree.

The National Leprosy Control Programme (NLCP) was launched in 1954-55. The pace of NLCP was slow during the first 25 years of its existence. The methodology followed was a mass campaign for early case-detection and bringing them under DDS treatment. It was supported by health-education activities with twin aims of reduction of quantum of infection in the community and interruption of transmission of disease to the healthy. The programme gained momentum from the IV Plan period onwards, after it was made into an entirely Centrally-sponsored scheme. But, by the end of IV Plan period only 1/3rd of endemic population was covered, which in subsequent V Plan made up to more than 3/4th of the endemic population coverage. The progress of case-detection, population coverage, quantum of expenditure and pattern of assistance in the Five Year Plans are summarised in Tables 6.2 and 6.3.

TABLE 6.2: Plan Expenditure, Population Coverage and Case-Detection of Leprosy Cases: I to V Plan

Period	Population covered (millions)	Cases detected & brought under treatment (million)	Expenditure (Rs. in millions)	Pattern of assistance
1st Plan (1951-56)	2.0	0.0017	3.500	Centrally aided
2nd Plan (1956-61)	14.51	0.112	52.900	Centrally aided
3rd Plan (1961-66)	15.20	0.560	42.500	Centrally aided
Annual Plan (1966-69)	14.20	0.778	6.300	Centrally aided
4th Plan (1969-74)	130.80	1.240	28.600	100%
5th Plan (1974-79)	324.00	2.150	202.300	50:50

TABLE 6.3: Plan Expenditure and Pattern of Assistance: VI to VIII Plan

(Rs. in millions)

Period	Expenditure	Pattern of Assistance
Annual Plan (1979-80)	23.200	50 : 50
6th Plan (1980-85)	400.443	100%
7th Plan (1985-90)	858.200	100%
8th Plan (1990-91)	222.554	100%
(1991-92)	228.000	100%

In 1981, the Government of India, considering that a stage has arrived when it should be possible to evolve a strategy for undertaking an Eradication Programme for Leprosy by the turn of the century, set up a 'Working Group on the Eradication of Leprosy' under the chairmanship of the noted Scientist and Planning Commission Member, Dr. M.S. Swaminathan (WGEL, 1982). The main objective given of this Working Group was to formulate an appropriate strategy for the purpose, taking advantage of the great advances in the Chemotherapy of Leprosy, the extended reach of mass media, the promise of recent medical research and other relevant factors.

The Terms of Reference of the Working Group were:

I. In working out the strategy and recommending a time-bound action programme, the Working Group will focus, among other things on the following aspects:

(a) Chemotherapy including indigenous production of anti-leprosy drugs;
(b) Sociological dimensions;
(c) Legal aspects;
(d) Delivery System;
(e) Role of Voluntary Sector;
(f) Health education;
(g) Medical education and medical research; and
(h) Rehabilitation.

II. The main thrust of the Action Programme should be to reduce the reservoir of infection in the community in the shortest possible time.

The Working Group after deliberating at length submitted its report in February 1982. The Chairman, Dr. M.S. Swaminathan, in his endorsing remarks observed that the conclusion of the Committee was that "a more of the same approach" with reference to the leprosy control strategy will not lead us to the desired goal. It is essential to continue the medical with the social and human aspects of the problem and view all of them in their totality. The most urgent need is the spread of the message that leprosy is now a curable disease and that there is no need to be afraid of it.

'The most challenging tasks lie in the field of early case-detection and interruption of the transmission cycle. Case-retention for the full period of treatment and post-treatment rehabilitation. The total eradication of leprosy is going to be difficult so long as slums and sub-human living conditions persist, unless a safe and effective vaccine becomes available.'

As an Integrated Action Plan, the working group devised a Milestone Chart (Appendix 25), enumerating the broad aims of programme thrust and design:

(a) *Mass Awareness and Participation in the Sixth Plan during the Remaining Period (1982-85)* — Getting leprosy accepted by the Society as any other disease for which cure is available through mass education, will be the major programme thrust.
(b) *Attack Phase* — Intensified Chemotherapy Campaign : Seventh Plan (1985-90).
(c) *Consolidation Phase* — Eighth and Ninth Plans (1990-2000).

An Institutional structure for policy, guidance, programme implementation and monitoring and evaluation at the National level at apex and at the executive level, by way of setting up of (a) National Commission for Eradication of Leprosy, and (b) National Leprosy Eradication Board, respectively, were suggested by the Group. The similar administrative set-up with sumptuous cooperative efforts of both the Government and the Voluntary non-governmental sector were suggested for the States. Outlining the various recommendations the Working Group felt confident that leprosy can largely become a problem of the past when we enter the 21st century, provided the measures the Group has suggested are adopted and prompt follow-up action taken.

Over the years separate NLEP staff has been created in the field to provide exclusively anti-leprosy services, and in this sense it is a vertical set-up. Keeping in view a large case-load in 1983, it was decided to extend MDT to leprosy cases in a phased manner, starting from very highly endemic districts first. The priorities for selection of the district were:

(i) Complete infrastructure in position in the district;
(ii) Adequate training of leprosy staff in MDT operation;
(iii) Rapid survey to detect the undetected cases; and
(iv) Screening of all recorded cases and preparation of individual case-cards.

In the beginning of 1983, two districts were extended MDT and by the end of March 1992, 135 districts in the hyperendemic (above 5/1000) areas were covered under MDT, covering nearly 75 per cent of the recorded leprosy cases, i.e., 1.5 to 1.6 million. Over a million leprosy cases have been discharged since 1985, as disease getting cured due to effective MDT implementation.

A summary of targets fixed and achievements made in respect of case-detection, treatment and discharge of cases, year-wise since 1980-81 to 1990-91, is summarised in Table 6.4. Targeted achievements under NLEP from 1991 to year 2001 in respect of existing leprosy cases, new cases, discharge due to cure, death or otherwise and net number of cases in the respective years is brought out in Table 6.5. Flow-chart (Appendix I) summarises the existing infrastructure under the NLEP at the Centre, States, district and field levels.

TABLE 6.4: Target Fixed and Achievement in Caste-detection Treatment and Discharge: Yearwise, 1980-81 to 1990-91

(Figure in Lakhs)

Year	Detection of Cases		Treatment of Cases		Discharge of Cases	
	Target	Achievement	Target	Achievement	Target	Achievement
1980-81	4.07	3.01	4.07	2.90	2.03	1.82
1981-82	4.07	3.67	4.07	3.47	2.03	2.59
1982-83	4.73	5.13	4.73	4.86	3.54	2.66
1983-84	4.77	4.82	4.77	4.56	3.25	2.84
1984-85	4.90	4.81	4.90	4.57	3.42	3.44
1985-86	3.82	4.77	3.82	4.50	3.74	4.46
1986-87	4.20	5.08	4.20	4.88	4.30	5.07
1987-88	4.20	5.19	4.20	4.99	5.03	5.74
1988-89	3.90	4.74	3.90	4.65	5.94	6.05
1989-90	3.50	4.66	3.50	4.62	6.55	6.69
1990-91	3.69	4.68	3.69	4.61	8.81	9.72
Total	45.85	50.56	45.85	48.61	48.64	51.08

Major Recommendations of the Working Group

1. Constitution of a National Leprosy Control Commission (NLCC), with the Prime Minister as its Chairman, for the guidance and surveillance of the leprosy eradication programme is recommended. A

National Leprosy Eradication Board (NLEB) vested with the powers of Government and with the Union Health Secretary as its Chairman, may be constituted to serve as the Executive Body responsible for the implementation of the plans and policies of NLCC. It is recommended that States where there is a high incidence of leprosy may also constitute such Policy Guidance and Implementation Bodies under the chairmanship of the Chief Minister and the State Health Secretary respectively.

TABLE 6.5: Targeted Achievements under NLEP by Years

(Figure in millions)

Year	No. of cases at the beginning of the year	New cases	Discharge due to cure, death or otherwise	No. of cases at the end of the year
1991	2.043	+0.45	-0.75	1.743
1992	1.743	+0.43	-0.72	1.453
1993	1.453	+0.40	-0.68	1.173
1994	1.173	+0.37	-0.65	0.893
1995	0.893	+0.35	-0.62	0.623
1996	0.623	+0.30	-0.60	0.323
1997	0.323	+0.25	-0.48	0.093
1998	0.093	+0.23	-0.20	0.073
1999	0.073	+0.15	-0.25	0.023
2000	0.023	+0.10	-0.12	0.003
2001	0.003	+0.10	-0.103	0.000

2. Continuation of the vertical structure of the leprosy control programme with administrative and technical strengthening and streamlining of the leprosy cells at the Central, State and district levels is considered essential.

3. A systematic case detection campaign is recommended in the high endemic districts, to begin with, to bring all the cases under

treatment within specified period of time in order to (i) drastically interrupt disease transmission resulting in a rapid decline in the incidence of the disease, and (ii) prevent further emergence of drug resistant leprosy.

The existing single-drug therapy by DDS alone should be supplemented by the one or more bactericidal drugs including rifampicin at least for the treatment of smear-positive or infectious type of cases, in the form of a campaign which is likely to achieve substantial control of the disease and constitute a step further towards its eradication. In order to undertake such a campaign on a massive scale, the ongoing Sixth Plan Leprosy Control Scheme needs to be speedily implemented to lay the necessary infrastructure in the field and to prepare the ground. Health education, population survey, mass communication, training of staff and welfare services to the patients should be geared up for the success of the campaign.

4. To attract and retain doctors in leprosy control service, creation of a special sub-cadre for leprosy service in the State Health Services is recommended.

5. It is recommended that the Voluntary Institutions engaged in leprosy work be strengthened and their functioning made easier by timely release of grant money. Where appropriate, the employees under the grant-in-aid schemes to voluntary institutions be paid salaries on par with their counterparts in Government service. Government should make the necessary funds available for this purpose to voluntary organisations.

6. Unless medical students are made to learn leprosy as a part of their curriculum, by including compulsory questions on leprosy in their examination, inadequate interest in leprosy work among doctors in service, and general medical practitioners, will continue. It is, therefore, recommended that the recommendations of the Mukhopadhyay Committee of the Medical Council of India on teaching of leprosy to undergraduate medical students be immediately implemented.

7. In order to ease the situation resulting from shortage or lack of a Medical Officer (MO) in many control units and for better supervision of control units, and also to provide incentives by way of promotion to meritorious paramedical field workers, it is recommended that senior Paramedical Workers (PMWs) with at least ten years' experience be given one year's intensive training in the basics of general and community medicine in a special training course, and

on successful completion of such training, posted as officers in charge of leprosy control units.

8. Legislative measures at the Central and State levels need to be initiated to repeal the Indian Lepers Act (1898) and amend suitably legislation based on out-dated and unscientific premises. Some pieces of legislation enacted on the basis of old concepts are derogatory to the interests of the leprosy patients and their basic rights as human beings.

9. To make the leprosy eradication campaign popular and acceptable to the people, a nationwide mass education campaign needs to be launched and pursued vigorously to educate people on the true facts about leprosy and to remove superstitions and wrong beliefs and the social stigma associated with leprosy. Software development for health communication should receive high priority.

10. Research efforts in vital areas like development of methods for early diagnosis, identification of individuals with higher risk of developing leprosy, *in vitro* culture of the leprosy bacillus, development of newer drugs and immunomodulators, development and testing of anti-leprosy vaccine, etc., deserve utmost priority. Existing research institutes and facilities should be strengthened to take these up.

11. During the eradication phase, it is recommended that the programme officer for leprosy in the Health Directorate be designated as Director of Leprosy Control with the rank of a Deputy Director General of Health Services. Similarly, the leprosy programme officers in the States should not hold ranks below that of a Deputy Director of Health Services. The leprosy control staff in the districts may be placed under the direct administrative control and discipline of the State Leprosy Officer.

12. While it is difficult to visualise the extent of additional financial requirements at this stage, since the layout and expansion of facilities to be created have to be done in phases, the National Leprosy Eradication Board should go into the details of funds needed, as the programme expands. The Working Group, however, recommends an interim budget covering the remaining years of the Sixth Plan period providing for the execution of the action plan for this period as outlined in the Milestone Chart (Appendix 25).

13. A National Consortium to coordinate the activities of all the voluntary organisations may be constituted. The Government can help such a body to raise funds from donors with the benefit of tax

exemption. A revolving fund created and controlled by the consortium may be utilised to help voluntary institutions in times of cash flow problems.

14. It will be useful if the Lok Sabha, Rajya Sabha and the State Legislatures pass resolutions endorsing eradication of leprosy by the end of this century as a national goal.

15. Intensive efforts need to be launched if India has to become self-sufficient in the requirement of anti-leprosy drugs. Till the indigenous production of these drugs reaches the required level, the additional quantities required will have to be obtained from external sources to meet the existing demand. The support of suitable bilateral and UN agencies could be enlisted for obtaining the needed drugs.

16. It is essential that rehabilitation becomes an integral part of leprosy control. For this purpose, coordinated efforts by the Departments of Health, Education and Social Welfare as well as voluntary organisations are necessary. The Ministry of Health and Family Welfare may function as the nodal point for this purpose. Leprosy colonies should be provided with the minimum basic needs of food, water, housing and work opportunities.

17. Incentives by way of cash and other means should be given to patients for prompt and regular drug consumption and attendance. Special "Food for Cure" programmes may also be introduced in areas characterised by a high prevalence of the disease.

18. Children of leprosy patients (and child patients of leprosy) should receive priority attention under the Integrated Child Development Services (ICDS).

19. Screening of pre-school children and youth for possible infection through "Skin Camps" should become a regular activity. The help of NSS and NCC students may be enlisted in such a mass case detection programme, after they are given appropriate training for this purpose. With proper preparation, this programme may be initiated during summer 1982.

20. "A more of the same approach" will not take us to the desired goal. What is needed is the integration of medical control methods with a human approach to the problem. Concern and compassion should permeate the control programme. The Milestone Chart suggested for the control programme indicates the order of priorities which may help us to reach the desired goal by the end of this century.

Introduction of MDT in NLEP

Due to limitation of dapsone monotherapy in the control of leprosy because of (i) prolonged treatment adversely effecting the case holding, and (ii) evidence of development of DDS resistance, the MDT was proposed to be introduced in all the 201 hyperendemic districts with prevalence rates of 5 or more per 1000 population as the national policy since 1983 (NLEP, 1987), in a phased manner for the treatment of all cases of leprosy, priority being given to MB patients.

The main objectives of MDT were:

(i) to render all infectious cases non-infectious in a short period so as to interrupt the chain of transmission of the disease in the community;
(ii) to give adequate and regular treatment to all the existing and new cases and cure them in a short period;
(iii) to prevent the emergence of drug resistant strain of M. leprae;
(iv) to ensure early detection and treatment of cases to prevent deformities;
(v) to carry out systemic health education activities with a view to disseminate important facts about leprosy and to remove social stigma; and
(vi) to prevent leprosy.

To ensure the satisfactory implementation of MDT in the district, both with regard to its quality and coverage, the following infrastructure was considered mandatory (Table 6.6):

(a) The entire population of the district should be covered by Leprosy Control Units (LCUs) and Urban Leprosy Centres (ULCs) in the ratio of one for every 400,000 of rural and 50,000 of urban population, respectively.
(b) The District Leprosy Officer (DLO) should be functioning in the district, supported by recommended ancillary staff.
(c) It is desirable that Temporary Hospitalisation Wards (THWs) are available in the district.
(d) The infrastructure envisaged at various levels as per schedule.
(e) The districts should have detected atleast 80 per cent of the estimated cases, evolve a system of regular treatment of the patients and also have a laboratory attached to each Unit.

TABLE 6.6: Basic Infrastructure for MDT Implementation

1. The infrastructure envisaged

At District Level:

District Leprosy Officer (DLO)	1
Health Educator	1
Non-medical Supervisor (NMS)	1
Para-medical Worker (PMW)	1
Laboratory Technician	1
Upper/Lower Division Clerk/Typist	2
Store Keeper*	1
Accountant	1
Statistical Assistant	1
Driver—1, Helper—1, Peon—1	1

Leprosy Control Unit (LCU)/Modified Control Unit (MCU)

Medical Officer (MO)	
Non-medical Supervisor – 1 per 100,000	
Para-medical Worker (PMW) – 1 per 15-25 thousands,	
Laboratory Technician	2
Physiotherapist	1
Health Educator*	1
Statistical Assistant*	1

Clerk—2, Driver—1, Peon—1, Sweeper—1, Helper—1

One LCU covers a population of 4 to 5 lacs. MCU would have less number of supervisory staff

At Urban Leprosy Centre – Upgraded Leprosy Centre

Medical Officer	1
Health Educator	1
Laboratory Technician	1
Non-medical Supervisor	1
Clerk—1, Driver—1, Peon—1	1

Other Urban Leprosy Centres:

Non-medical Supervisor	1
Survey, Education and Treatment Centre	1
Para-medical Worker	1

2. To finance the above items it is proposed to establish a Society for each of the MDT district to be taken up under NLEP to be registered under the Societies Registration Act with the following composition:

(a) Collector/Dy. Commissioner/Chief Executive Officer, Zilla Parishad	—Chairman
(b) Chief District Medical Officer	—Vice-Chairman
(c) State Leprosy Officer	—Member
(d) Consultant Leprologist	—Member

(e) District Education or Social Welfare Officer —Member

(f) Representative of the Local Voluntary Organisation Involved in Leprosy —Member

(g) District Leprosy Officer/Secretary —Member

3. The society will be responsible to oversee the implementation of the Programme and directly financing the above items. The grant-in-aid admissible will be as per the terms of modified MDT which will be sanctioned to the Society so constituted. The Society will be fully responsible for utilisation of these grant-in-aids as per terms and will render accounts to the Government of India as prescribed. The Society will also decide the payment of awards to the patients for taking complete treatment in schedule time in cash or kind not exceeding Rs. 100 per patient.
4. As there may be more than one local voluntary organisation working under the leprosy field in a particular district, the representative of the voluntary organisation on the Society may be nominated by rotation. The representative of the voluntary organisation so nominated must, however, be resident of the district.
5. An accounting procedure to be followed for financing the above components of modified MDT has been formulated and the same will be circulated alongwith revised guidelines.
6. The State Governments are requested to take immediate action to constitute the societies in each district to be taken up under modified MDT scheme and have them registered under the Societies Registration Act within one month of issue of sanction. The Memorandum and Articles of Association of the societies in the MDT districts may be drawn up and a copy thereof sent to the Government of India alongwith the intimation about the constitution of the societies under the Societies Registration Act. The District Leprosy Officer may be asked to apply for the grant-in-aid in accordance with the prescribed proforma which will be sanctioned direct to him to ensue speedy implementation of the programme.

---

* Optional

The MDT project was implemented in the selected endemic districts in the following four phases:

(i) Mobilisation Phase;
(ii) Planning and Preparatory Phase;
(iii) Intensive Phase; and
(iv) Maintenance Phase.

(i) *Mobilisation Phase*

In the Mobilisation Phase following activities were required to be carried out:

(a) Positioning of staff members in accordance with pattern of deployment and provisions of physical infrastructure, e.g., vehicles, laboratory facilities, referral institution, etc.
(b) Providing basic training to untrained staff members.
(c) Conducting surveys to detect at least 80 per cent of the total estimated cases should be completed.
(d) Involving other health staff including Multipurpose Workers (MPWs) by imparting suitable orientation.

The satisfactory completion of this phase should be reviewed and approved by the State Coordination Committee before the next phase commences.

(ii) *Planning and Preparatory Phase*

Following activities are mendatory for this phase:

(a) At least one rapid survey must be conducted in the district so as to detect the remaining 20 per cent of estimated cases, as per guidelines issued by the Government of India (Appendix 11).
(b) Sample surveys should be carried out by the epidemiological assessment team, independent of the DLO, in the first year of the preparatory phase and shall be repeated at yearly intervals.
(c) Screening of all the identified cases must be done by the medical officer personally for each and every case. With a view to classify the cases as MB/PB, initial BI, preparing the individual case-card, all inactive cases, etc. should be listed out.
(d) Specific plan of operation for Intensive Phase (Phase iii) regarding circuit plan of drug delivery is required to be prepared by the DLO in consultation with State Leprosy Officer (SLO) and the Programme Coordinator, Government of India, as per Appendix 11.
(e) Training of the remaining newly posted workers at all levels by an intensive, short term orientation of 3-5 days on MDT and its implementation.

(f) Laboratory attached to each unit will be improved to effectively monitor the BI in MB cases.

(iii) *Intensive Phase*

On satisfactory completion of the Planning and Preparatory Phase (Phase ii) as approved by the State Coordination Committee, a district will enter into Intensive Phase during which:

(a) A systematic and scientific implementation of MDT will be carried out up to three years with the financial support of the Central Government or any other agency identified by it.
(b) MDT will be completed for the known cases as well as for most of the new cases identified during the first two years within the schedule period of three years.
(c) After the intensive daily treatment for 14 days is over in all circuits in a control unit, half the number of days in each month will be needed for drug delivery by circuits for pulse treatment and the remaining days can be utilised for new case-detection by school surveys, contact and general population surveys in the area so that, within this period of 3 years, one more round of screening of the population is carried out.
(d) Health-education activities, rehabilitation aspects of leprosy patients and their families and supportive activities relevant to the prevention and control of leprosy will be promoted. Periodic monitoring of operational and epidemiological aspects will continue, culminated by a mid-term and final evaluation of the project.

(iv) *Maintenance Phase*

After the Intensive Phase (Phase iii), the Maintenance Phase will commence and continue for five years during this Phase:

(a) Newly detected patients in the community or immigrant cases will be treated so that all the potential sources of infection in the community are brought under MDT. With increasing cure rate the incidence of disease is likely to decline and the number of new cases will become less due to interruption in the transmission of the disease; and

(b) PHC staff would be involved in leprosy control activities in phases so that they takeover the left over responsibilities of the programme at the end of this phase.

The successful implementation of MDT in 136 hyperendemic districts out of 201 such districts with more than 5/1000 prevalence proved that MDT is a sure method of elimination of leprosy from endemic countries under the circumstances. It has succeeded in bringing down the total case load from 4 million to around 2.7 million by late 1990. But in spite of such success with all the perseverance and drive on the part of programme managers and committed political will, the programme could be brought to execution in only 136 hyperendemic districts, and 66 such districts still remained uncovered.

The reasons for it were not far to seek. The vertical programme necessary was high cost-operative and required a select group of intensively trained medical infrastructure exclusively meant to run it. The intensive therapy schedule of every day 600 mg Rifampicin for first 14 days in cases of MB MDT were further impediment in spreading the programme more extensively.

At the end of 1990, due to drastic reduction in prevalence and new case-detection rate and release from treatment and surveillance of a large number of treated and cured patients, eleven such hyperendemic districts are proposed for integration with general health care set-up (Appendix 4) and other 125 districts covered under regular MDT (Appendix 2) may follow suit.

Realising the need to cover the vast population under MDT and no longer keeping them deprived of the effective tool of eradication of the leprosy, Director General of Health Services to the Government of India, observed:

> 'Leprosy Control is based on appropriate treatment delivery. Hence, it is all the more necessary to remember, when we are planning for MDT, as to what is expected of us by the leprosy patients who are not receiving treatment. Our first job is to start them on MDT without any more delay. The services, which provide MDT, must have a wide coverage to reach every part of the country. It must be able to maintain regular and frequent contact with the patients and the community. A District Health System based on Primary Health Care (PHC) is more or less self-

contained segment of national health delivery system. It is important to recognise that MDT could be and should be implemented through existing general health care system.

Though 130 out of 196 endemic districts have been brought under MDT, the major concern is how to bring quickly the remaining 66 problem districts under MDT. The problem has been accentuated due to lack of trained manpower and large uncovered areas. It is time to involve PHC for MDT delivery. . .'

Modified MDT Scheme

The conventional MDT (as modified by Indian Leprologists) could, by late 1990, cover only 130 out of 196 endemic districts with 283 million population and 2.1 million leprosy cases, constituting 65-68 per cent of the recorded leprosy cases. Out of the remaining leprosy patients, nearly 25 per cent cases are from the 66 endemic districts (Appendix 3) majority (56) of them being in the States of Madhya Pradesh, Uttar Pradesh, Bihar, Orissa, Kerala and West Bengal. Most of these districts have inadequate infrastructure to implement MDT as per Government of India guidelines (Appendix 11) issued for endemic districts. At the same time, it is essential to extend the benefit of MDT to the patients in these districts without further delay to achieve the target of arresting the disease by 2000 AD.

The endemic districts, where it is not possible/feasible to create vertical set-up by March 3, 1991, the revised strategy of extension of MDT with existing staff, including primary health care will be introduced (NLEP, 1990a).

Each endemic district under Modified MDT Scheme would have a registered District Leprosy Society under the chairmanship of District Collector, with Chief Medical Officer of the district as Vice-Chairman and DLO as Member-Secretary responsible for operating the funds under the project.

The main objectives of the Modified MDT Programme are:

(a) To render all infectious cases as non-infectious in a short period so as to interrupt the chain of transmission of the disease in the community;
(b) To give adequate and regular treatment to all the existing and new cases and cure them in a short period;

(c) To prevent the emergence of drug resistant strains of M. Leprae;
(d) To ensure early detection and treatment of cases to prevent deformities;
(e) To carry out systematic health education activities, with a view to disseminate important facts about leprosy and to remove social stigma;
(f) To prevent the spread of leprosy; and
(g) To finally eradicate leprosy.

Differences in Technical Content of Modified MDT Scheme

The main points of difference in the Modified MDT Scheme *vis-à-vis* MDT are:

(a) Fourteen days intensive therapy for MB cases will be discontinued.
(b) Fixed duration of chemotherapy will be introduced for MB and PB cases. However, PB with multiple lesions will be examined at the time of sixth pulse.
(c) Instead of rapid survey prescribed in the Government of India existing guidelines (Appendix 11), Health Education Activities will be intensified to encourage voluntary reporting. It is expected that adequate case detection can be ensured by intensive Health Education supported by screening and patient satisfaction due to effective treatment.
(d) Bacteriological examination of skin smears will be confined to MB cases and suspected MB cases. However, MDT will be started on basis of clinical examination.

On the operative side the Modified MDT Scheme envisages to introduce:

(a) A scheme of awards for PHC functionaries based on their performance. The details of the Scheme to be worked out separately.
(b) To improve new case detection, an incentive of Rs. 3 per new case detected/reported.
(c) Payment of Rs. 10 to the patient for each supervised pulse administered, limiting 24 pulses in MB and 6 pulses in PB to

improve case holding. In addition patients taking the full course in prescribed period will get Rs. 100 in cash or kind as may be decided by the District Leprosy Society.

Role of VOs/NGOs in National Leprosy Eradication

Long before the governmental effort, the leprosy work was undertaken in the missionary spirit way back in 19th century in India by way of establishment of 'leper' asylums at Calcutta, Varanasi and Chamba. The British Empire Leprosy Relief Association (precursor of Hind Kusht Nivaran Sangh or Indian Leprosy Association) in 1925 laid the foundations of organised leprosy work in India. Since 1951 extensive expansion in voluntary organisations (VOs) for leprosy work has taken place and at present about 285 VOs are actively engaged in leprosy relief work.

Some of the VOs (NLEP, 1988) engaged in leprosy work are:

(A) International

(a) World Health Organisation
(b) UNICEF
(c) Leprosy Mission
(d) German Leprosy Relief Association
(e) Damien Foundation, Brussels
(f) International Federation of Anti-Leprosy Association (ILEP)

(B) National

(i) Gandhi Memorial Leprosy Foundation
(ii) Many other organisations working in various parts of the country.

These VOs are helping in:

(i) Patient Care;
(ii) Surveys;
(iii) Health-education;
(iv) Rehabilitation;
(v) Training of Medical and Para-medical Personnel; and
(vi) Referral Centres.

(vi) Referral Centres.

With a bed strength of 14,409 in 1990, 127 VOs have vocationally rehabilitated 35,275 leprosy affected persons and nearly 20,000 persons have been medically treated.

The VOs are increasingly working in cooperation with NLEP with the common objective of eradication the disease by 2000.

Training Facilities

Forty-nine Leprosy Training Centres throughout the country train the medical and para-medical personnel engaged in leprosy eradication work. So far 550 medical officers and 21,220 para-medical workers have been trained since 1955. But still a shortfall of trained medical as well as para-medical personnel exists in the programme. The working of the Training Centres has been reviewed by a Committee of experts set up by DGHS in 1986-87. Following activities have been recommended.

(a) A training cell be created at Directorate General of Health Services (DGHS) under Leprosy Division to provide for specific requisite planning, implementation and follow-up of staffing and their training needs.
(b) Orientation training of short duration for the general health care staff should be considered necessary.

Health Education Activities in MDT Districts

For promoting leprosy control activities and their acceptance by the people, it is essential to have a plan of action for carrying out health education utilising various mass media to impart knowledge on the following crucial facts about leprosy:

(i) Leprosy is not a curse or past sin;
(ii) It is not hereditary;
(iii) It is the least infectious of all communicable diseases;
(iv) It can be completely cured at any stage; and
(v) Early detection and regular treatment will prevent deformities.

The actual media selected may vary from area to area, but in general, all available audio-visual media, viz., radio, television, wall paintings, hoardings, rickshaw and bus boards, and the like, cinema slides, advertisements, films, exhibition, etc., will be fully exploited to carry the messages of health education.

Recommended Orientation Training Activities

For the effective implementation of MDT for leprosy, adequate training of various participating members of the team is very essential.

The schedule of training for various groups of personnel under NLEP is shown in Table 6.7.

TABLE 6.7: Schedule of Training for NLEP Staff

NLEP Staff requiring training in the district	Duration	Place
1. Medical Officers including general health cadre	7 days	to be specified by District Leprosy Officer
2. Non-Medical Supervisor	7 days	
3. Laboratory Technicians	7 days	
4. Para-medical Workers	7 days	Leprosy Training Centre of institution or the place specified by DLO
5. Health Educators	7 days	
6. Physio-technicians	5 days	
7. All Other General Staff Cadre	5 days	

Training Programme in Modified MDT Scheme of NLEP

I. *Medical Officers (PHC)* — The objective of the training programme is that, at the end of four days training, the Medical Officer incharge of the PHC will be able to:

(i) Manage a leprosy control programme;
(ii) Diagnose and classify a case of leprosy;
(iii) Treat leprosy;
(iv) Identify and treat complications;
(v) Prevent disabilities;
(vi) Organise Community Education Programme on Leprosy;

(vii) Document and prepare appropriate reports; and
(viii) Impart knowledge about how to train MPW on leprosy.

(a) To achieve the above objectives, the course outline as shown in Table 6.8 will be adopted:

TABLE 6.8: Course Outline for Training of Medical Officer (PHC)

Skill	Knowledge	Hours
1. Management of Leprosy-Control Programme	Know the epidemiology of leprosy, basis of leprosy control/NLEP.	3
2. Diagnose and classify a case of leprosy	a. Know the cardinal signs of leprosy. b. Know the systematic set. Procedure to be followed in screening a person for leprosy. c. Recognise the various types of leprosy. d. Identify various clinical manifestations. e. Record the clinical findings in a suitable form for subsequent monitoring of progress. f. Know various other skin diseases which simulate leprosy lesions.	6
3. To Treat leprosy	a. Anti-leprosy drugs. b. Drug Regimens. c. Side effects. d. MDT implementation.	2
4. Identify and treat complications	a. Clinical features of lepra reactions. b. Consequences. c. Anti-reaction drugs and management.	2
5. Prevention of disabilities	a. Know pre-disposing factors. b. Appropriate measures to prevent disabilities. c. Management of early disabilities. d. Protective aids. e. Physio-therapy. f. Health Education (HE)	2
6. Community Education	a. Methods of HE b. Organise HE Programmes.	1
7. Documentation	a. Know various indicators. b. How to calculate these indicators. c. Uses of these indicators. d. NLEP reporting format.	1
8. Evaluation	Pre- and Post-test	1

(b) Utilising various audio-visual teaching aids four-day schedule of teaching as given in Table 6.9 will be adopted.

TABLE 6.9: Training Programme on Leprosy for Medical Officer (PHC): Modified MDT Scheme of NLEP

	8.30-9.30	9.30-10.30	10.30-11.00	11.00-12.00	12.00-1.30	1.30-2.30	2.30-3.00	3.00-4.00
Day 1	Pre-test Introduction	Epidemiology	Coffee Break	Diagnosis Case taking 1/2	Lunch Break	Diagnosis Case taking 2/2	Coffee Break	Class and Cli.Mani 1/3
Day 2	Class and Clin.Mani 2/3	Reaction 1/2	Coffee Break	Reaction 2/2	Lunch Break	Differential Diagnosis	Coffee Break	Cli.Mani 3/3
Day 3	Leprosy Control	Disability Prevention 1/2	Coffee Break	Disability Prevention 2/2	Lunch Break	Health Education	Coffee Break	Indicators
Day 4	Modified NLEP	MDT 1/2	Coffee Break	MDT 2/2	Lunch Break	Evaluation Post test	Coffee Break	

Notes: (i) 1/3 of the Clinical Subject sessions should be devoted to Case Demonstrations.
(ii) Maximum usage of all possible teaching aids is recommended.
(iii) Class = Classification.
(iv) Cli Mani = Clinical Manifestation.

II. Multi-purpose Health Workers are to be given a highly condensed two-day course on various aspects of leprosy, at PHC level with a view to integrate the Vertical Leprosy Programme (VLP) to the PHC. The training programme has been planned in the form of 5 modules — each module relating to a particular aspect of leprosy related activity. They are:

Module 1 : Clinical and epidemiological aspects of leprosy.
Module 2 : Drug treatment of leprosy and management of complications.
Module 3 : Prevention of disability and care of anaesthetic limbs.
Module 4 : Community education.
Module 5 : NLEP/Modified MDT Programme/Health Workers' role in the same.

A suggested time-table of activities for a two-day training programmes is given in Table 6.10.

TABE 6.10: Time-table of Two-day Training Programme

Day	Time	Subject
First	08.00 - 09.30	Clinical and epidemiological aspects
	10.00 - 11.30	Clinical and epidemiological aspects
	11.30 - 12.30	Drug Treatment, Management of Complications
	14.00 - 15.00	Drug Treatment, Management of Complications
	15.30 - 16.30	Drug Treatment, Management of Complications
Second	08.00 - 10.00	Prevention of disability
	10.30 - 12.30	Community education
	14.00 - 15.30	NLEP, Modified MDT Programme, Local logistics
	16.00 - 16.30	Final Session : Evaluation, Questions and Answers clarification of doubts, etc.

Independent Evaluation of NLEP

Since 1986, NLEP is being jointly evaluated by the Government of India and World Health Organisation in alternate years. The last such Evaluation was conducted by a Team of National and International Experts in December 1991 (NLEP, 1991). The terms of reference for the last Independent Evaluation Team (IET) were:

1. To assess the effectiveness of the various operational activities relating to the Programme at the unit, district and State levels, including:

   (a) detection of new cases and discharge of inactive patients;
   (b) reliability of diagnosis and disease classification;
   (c) regularity of drug intake and reasons for default;
   (d) dependability of laboratory services.

2. To assess the utilisation of infrastructural facilities.
3. To validate the reported data through personal observation in the field and examination of records.
4. To assess the impact of HE in the community.
5. To assess the adequacy of information reporting system.
6. To assess the preparedness of modified MDT districts for initiating programme activities.
7. To examine the provision/creation of infrastructural facilities and ascertain the reasons for shortfall, if any.
8. To submit a report with collected data and make suitable recommendations on its basis.

The 15 Evaluation Teams visited 5-7 districts each, covering 24 of the States/UTs in the country from December 10 to 19 December, 1991. The districts covered were of all hues, viz., non-MDT, MDT, Modified MDT. The MDT districts were brought under MDT at various periods of time in the past.

The Evaluation Teams screened the enclosed data base of NLEP (Table 6.11), and interviewed a large number of respondents (Table 6.12).

Important Observations of the IV Evaluation Teams

1. The new case detection, MDT coverage and release from treatment were by and large considered satisfactory, except for the fact that case-detection should further be activated through mass surveys, school surveys and house-to-house patient search.
2. Untrained staff in sufficient numbers existed within the Programme while the training facilities remained grossly underutilised.

TABLE 6.11: Fourth Independent Evaluation of NLEP Data Base

Parameters	Number
States/UTs	24
Districts	77
Urban Leprosy Centres	16
Leprosy Control Units	83
Modified Leprosy Control Units	4
Survey, Education and Treatment Centres	3
Primary Health Centres	19
Sample Survey and Assessment Units	10
Leprosy Training Centres	11
Villages	88
Voluntary Organisations	29

TABLE 6.12: Fourth Independent Evaluation of NLEP Respondents Interviewed

Categories	Number
States Leprosy officers	24
DLOs/MOs	198
Non-Medical Supervisors	174
Laboratory Technicians	98
Para-medical Workers	167
Multipurpose Workers	15
Physio-therapists/Physio-technicians	34
Health Educators	41
Community Members	424
Patients	466

3. The Programme suffered from significant number of vacancies at each level, specially, with regard to physio-therapists, laboraroty technicians and health educators.
4. Temporary hospital wards were under-utilised.
5. Bacteriological surveillance continued to remain a weak link in the chain in the Programme.
6. The Sample Survey-cum-Assessment Units (SSAUs) should be looked into both in respect to their staffing and work-load with a view to attending to needs of finding out true disease prevalence in areas which were surveyed decades back and to conducting fresh surveys in so-called low-endemic areas in a phased manner.

7. Integration of leprosy services with PHC and Modified MDT scheme were beset with problems. They needed to be looked into immediately and carefully.
8. The non-endemic areas have remained in relative neglect and extension of MDT to these should be considered expeditiously.

The NLEP has made a definite impact on the curative aspects of leprosy patients in the hyperendemic districts (prevalence more than 5/1000 population) under the vertical set-up implementation. This is evident from the fact that by March 1991, 20,43,136 patients of leprosy were on record, 18,77,199 were brought under treatment and 54,15,884 were discharged from treatment after completion of MDT (Table 6.13). The cause for concern has remained in the hyper-endemic districts where MDT could not be so far implemented (66 districts) and which are now to be brought under Modified MDT scheme in partial integration with PHC system. The introduction of Modified MDT is besieged with many problems, the most important of them being:

(i) Insufficient training component of PHC staff, both medical and paramedical personnel.
(ii) Bringing in of monetary component, in respect of (i) payment to health personnel who bring in the newly detected cases under treatment, and (ii) inducement to the patient concerned for 6 to 24 monthly visits, in cases of pauci- and multi-bacillary types of leprosy, respectively.
(iii) Inadequate emphasis on laboratory component, e.g., BI testing.

In spite of all the serious efforts and inputs the programme has remained operative in the hyperendemic districts only so far and moderately and low-endemic districts, i.e., below 5/1000 prevalence have remained untouched to a large measure. After proven efficacy of MDT as a line of treatment for leprosy there is no justification whatsoever for continuing with monotherapy with DDS and monetary and administrative wherewithal is to be provided on utmost priority basis, otherwise, we are giving an opportunity for DDS resistance and number of leprosy cases to multiply in the community.

TABLE 6.13: Total Number of Leprosy Cases on Record, under Treatment and Discharged by States as on March 1991

Sl. No.	State/U.T.	Cases on record	Cases under treatment	Cases discharged
1.	Andhra Pradesh	214235	214235	1190031
2.	Arunachal Pradesh	1301	1301	813
3.	Assam	18766	18446	13179
4.	Bihar	462710	418689	264080
5.	Goa	1245	1245	3917
6.	Gujarat	24901	24864	128230
7.	Haryana	1282	1282	918
8.	Himachal Pradesh	3957	3957	3299
9.	J & K	6356	5456	1873
10.	Karnataka	39470	39470	263859
11.	Kerala	65817	53544	79209
12.	Madhya Pradesh	159850	124598	188864
13.	Maharashtra	166619	166619	839561
14.	Manipur	1365	1365	4667
15.	Meghalaya	1394	1394	1199
16.	Mizoram	201	193	680
17.	Nagaland	2030	2030	583
18.	Orissa	157621	156966	330106
19.	Punjab	3291	2991	4651
20.	Rajasthan	15549	13961	8026
21.	Sikkim	225	225	248
22.	Tamil Nadu	207116	202897	1171891
23.	Tripura	2706	2706	2446
24.	Uttar Pradesh	361568	316939	368712
25.	West Bengal	114349	92974	529566
26.	A & N Island	1347	1347	1243
27.	Chandigarh	936	878	13
28.	D & N Haveli	383	368	64
29.	Daman & Diu	192	192	96
30.	Delhi	4232	3945	1097
31.	Lakshadweep	159	159	443
32.	Pondicherry	1963	1963	12320
	Total	2043136	1877199	5415884

The Research is an another area which has not received the due priority as it should have been. This had been true both with the testing of newer anti-leprosy drugs and the role of various vaccines in immunoprophylaxis and as an adjunct to the available chemotherapy in the matter of early clearance of granuloma and reduction of BI.

So far the health administrators' concern had been on only reducing the number of infective bacilliferous cases in the community without sufficient care for the disabled and concern for the rehabilitative aspects of the cases discharged from treatment.

REFERENCE

Dharmendra, 1978, *Leprosy*, Kothari Medical Publishing, House, Bombay, vol. 1, p. 27

NLEP, 1987, *Guideline for Multidrug Treatment in Endemic Districts*, revised edition, Leprosy Division, Directorate General of Health Services, New Delhi.

NLEP, 1988, *Voluntary Organisations in Leprosy Eradication*, Leprosy Division, Directorate General of Health Services, New Delhi.

NLEP, 1990a, *Guidelines for Modified MDT Scheme in Selected Districts*, Leprosy Division, Directorate of Health Services, New Delhi.

NLEP, 1990b, *Training Manual for Medical Officers and Health Supervisors*, Leprosy Division, Directorate General of Health Services, New Delhi.

NLEP, 1990c, *Training Manual for Health Workers*, Leprosy Division, Directorate General of Health Services, New Delhi.

NLEP, 1990d, *Background Material Issued to IV Independent Evaluation Teams*, Leprosy Division, Directorate General of Health Services, New Delhi.

NLEP, 1991, *IV Independent Evaluation, 1991*, Leprosy Division, Directorate General of Health Services, New Delhi.

WGEL, 1982, *Report of the Working Group on the Eradication of Leprosy, February, 1982*, Leprosy Division, Directorate General of Health Services, New Delhi.

WHSQ, 1991, *World Health Statistics Quarterly*, Vol. 44, No. 1.

7

EVALUATION OF LEPROSY CONTROL MEASURES IN SOME LOW-ENDEMIC AREAS OF INDIA

7.1 LEPROSY SITUATION IN NORTH EASTERN REGION OF INDIA WITH SPECIAL REFERENCE TO ASSAM, MEGHALAYA AND TRIPURA

R. GANAPATI, ATUL C. SHAH and THOMAS ABRAHAM

Leprosy control efforts of National Leprosy Eradication Programme (NLEP) with multi-drug therapy (MDT), in most regions of the country over the past decade, has been praiseworthy, as the prevalence of the so-called active cases has come down remarkably in many districts especially Southern regions of the country. However, in many endemic districts in North Indian States the programme has not been successful. North Eastern States,* traditionally believed to have low endemicity, have even received much less attention. The authors had an opportunity of visiting three States in this regions, namely, Assam, Meghalaya and Tripura, as members of the IV Independent Evaluation Team (IET) of NLEP in the month of December 1991. Some of the observations gathered during this visit and some suggestions and recommendations for effective eradication of disease are presented.

Monotherapy with Diamino-diphenyl Sulphone (DDS) is still practised in most of the States, though in some patches MDT is attempted. Impressions summarised here, it is believed, would generally be applicable to almost all monotherapy States.

---

* The North-Eastern region comprises seven States, viz., Arunachal Pradesh, Assam, Meghalaya, Manipur, Mizoram, Nagaland and Tripura.

Assam

Assam is the largest State in this region with an area of 78,438 sq km with a population of 2.2 crores. Guwahati is the capital city with a hilly terrain, dense rain forests and green paddy fields characterising the rural scenario.

Total number of leprosy cases under treatment is 18,815 with registered prevalence rate of 0.81 per thousand. The estimated prevalence rate is 1.48 per thousand.

The places IET visited, mostly in Kamrup and Navgaon districts, were (1) Leprosy Training Centre (LTC), Boko; (2) Temporary Hospitalization Ward (THW), Boko; (3) Leprosy Asylum, Boko; (4) Reconstructive Surgery Unit (RSU), Boko; (5) Assam Seva Samiti, Titlia; (6) Upgraded Urban Leprosy Control Centre (ULC), Guwahati Medical College, Guwahati; (7) Survey, Education, Treatment (SET) Unit, and Primary Health Centre (PHC), Panpur; (8) SET Centre, Azara; and (9) SET Centre, Nelli State Dispensary, Navgaon.

The SET programme in the State is not effective. The centre visited by the team revealed that the work is sluggish and manned by medical officer-in-charge of State Health Dispensary, whose knowledge about leprosy, especially aspects relating to treatment is even poorer than the non-medical assistant (NMA) working under him. Surveys seem to be carried out by NMA, but confirmation of cases is unsatisfactory and number of patients handled by NMA is very low.

Terrain, weather, paucity of vehicles and absence of trained survey teams affect the detection of new cases leading to false positive low prevalence rate. Majority of patients are on monotherapy.

Reliability of the registered patients, diagnosis and disease classification, however, is reasonably satisfactory, inspite of the fact that the majority of staff is untrained or partly trained. The laboratory services are extremely poor. With all the deficiencies,the reported data and the records, however, seem to give some information, which could help better planning of the programme in future.

LTC at Boko can hardly be termed as a training centre. Buildings and staff are grossly under-utilised and there are practically no trained personnel. However, for the North Eastern region, LTC is the only centre offering some hope because of the existence of some basic infrastructural facilities including THW and RSU, which are at present non-functional. In THW there are florid lepromatous (histoid) cases and rare varieties of the disease – the types which have become exceedingly rare even in hyperendemic areas where MDT is available freely (Fig. 7.1.1). The key to leprosy control in North Eastern region could possibly be the total revamping and revitalising of this centre.

A very significant factor is the interest shown by the voluntary organisations (VOs), e.g., Assam Sewa Samiti Shankar Mission, although there are not many VOs in the State. As it is well known, the benefits of VOs in the country have been perceptible more in endemic regions, especially South India, and there has been a distinct neglect by VOs in such low prevalent zones. Assam could be cited as an example of such a neglect. Involvement of VOs and the coordination of the governmental and voluntary activity to achieve the NLEP objective is now an established fact. The VOs in Assam are plagued by lack of finances, manpower and proper guidance on how to organise work in low endemic areas, as also procedural knowledge required to get grants and cooperation of the health services. VOs work reveals an element of isolation without coordination with the government agencies.

A redeeming feature in the State is the interest shown by the medical college staff, especially dermatologists, in academic matters pertaining to leprosy. However, they do not seem to work in cooperation with the agencies engaged in field work. They look at the problem mainly from the clinical angle.

Meghalaya

The terrain in Meghalaya is difficult and challenging. Here the actual prevalence rate (PR) of leprosy is reported to be 0.57 per thousand with an estimated PR of 3.4 per thousand (sample survey year not known). Most of the inactive cases are not released from treatment and it is difficult to determine the exact PR. The IET visited (1) Jowai Centre, Jaintia Hills district; (2) Unden Leprosy Control Unit (LCU) and THW, East Khashi Hills district; and (3) Mother Teresa Leprosy Charity House, a VO in East Khashi Hills.

The work in Meghalaya, which is mostly hilly and which has trained staff, is even worse than that in Assam. Survey is reported to have been carried out, but the case confirmation is extremely unreliable, though the classification in some advanced cases could seem to be acceptable. At some places one encounters an anomalous situation of LCU having 31 workers for a patient load of 42 and still showing more than 30 per cent defaulter rate. The laboratory services are as deplorable as those in Assam. Most of the staff has not been in position. THW has still not started functioning in full swing, though the infrastructure is fair and motivation of some senior staff is encouraging. State commitment for leprosy control work is wanting.

It is worth stressing here that Mother Teresa Leprosy Charity House is the only VO of its kind in the region where a large number of progressive leprosy patients are admitted and offered MDT. Some of the patients seem to come from outside the State. While the motivation in the institution is generally good, coordination between the staff of VO and Government needs strengthening; and this applies to all VOs.

Tripura

Tripura is a small State in the country. Hills and valleys constitute the total area of 10,491 sq km Population according to 1991 Census was 27.75 lakhs, 30 per cent of which are tribals.

IET, besides having discussions with health officials including the Health Minister, visited the following places in West Tripura district: (1) Office of the Zonal Leprosy Officer and LCU; (2) ULC, GB Hospital; and (3) Department of Dermatology, GB Hospital.

In contrast to the monotherapy States elsewhere in the North Eastern region, the situation in Tripura, due to effective implementation of MDT over the years, presented a refreshingly different picture. The staff working in LCU is quite competent and follows MDT guidelines systematically. Laboratory services, however, require strengthening. As no physiotherapist is available in West Tripura, disability care is not existent, and as such a physio-therapist is required to be provided.

ULC, being situated in a general hospital and attended by a dermatologist, is functioning well, though laboratory services are poor. There is motivation for disability care arising from trained orthopaedic surgeon, thereby emphasising the need for establishing an RSU in the campus. Two THWs, sanctioned for the North and South Tripura districts, are non-functional.

There are no VOs working exclusively for leprosy eradication in the whole State of Tripura.

Observations and Suggestions

The North Eastern region in the country, by and large, presents a pathetic situation, resulting from years of unmonitored administration of monotherapy in a difficult hilly terrain characterised by difficult logistics — the management being in the hands of untrained and partially trained, though somewhat motivated staff, with poor commitment on the part of the State Government, except in patchy areas where MDT is in vogue. Tripura State, due to fairly effective implementation of MDT through trained staff over the years, presents a far better picture.

Official prevalence maps (Figs. 7.1.2 and 7.1.3) show a distinct change in North Eastern region in general, though one should not be complacent about the clinical situation in this region.

Following suggestions are made under the assumption that, though arising from observations in three out of seven States, these may be applicable to the whole region as such:

1. Re-training of staff trained in the Monotheraphy era and training of untrained staff should be immediately undertaken.
2. Maximum advantage should be taken of the keen interest shown by medical institutions and medical colleges especially by dermatologists. Such institutions should be made important nucleus for leprosy activities in these States.
3. Lack of coordination of the functions of such institutions and the Directorate of Health Services, noticeable at present, should be rectified.
4. Teaching the staff and students of medical colleges, in particular, will have to be reoriented by periodical visits by experts from outside the State.
5. Maximum advantage should be taken of the motivation and the interest evinced by the government staff in leprosy work should be channelised to maximum advantage by conducting workshop-cum-training courses as frequently as possible with resource persons from reputed leprosy institutions elsewhere.
6. Rudimentary laboratory facilities, currently available in a patchy fashion, should be strengthened.
7. VOs, which show interest in academic work, (e.g., Assam Seva Samiti, Shankar Mission, Mother Teresa Leprosy Charity House, etc.) should be encouraged and guided to follow scientific line of treatment so that greater coordination with the government programme could be achieved.

8. The only LTC in Boko, which is catering for the whole of North Eastern region, should be revamped and revitalised, making use of the excellent infrastructural facilities like land, buildings, etc. The total ignorance of the staff, working especially in LTC is untenable. Training courses for trainers should be immediately arranged.
9. State Leprosy Councils, consisting of leprosy experts from outside the State, should be formed to advise the respective governments.
10. In States, where MDT is in progress, the staff should receive further training and encouragement so that they continue to work for leprosy eradication. Their expertise may be used to a greater extent elsewhere in monotherapy areas.
11. Guidance to staff in MDT districts from experts on management of relapses and residual problems after MDT is a necessity.
12. Working of the THWs and RSUs should be thoroughly overhauled and galvanised.
13. Disability care, as in most parts of the country, is still either non-existent or is in its infancy in the North Eastern region. Latest information and knowledge on offering care at the field level to prevent disability should be introduced gradually, and this requires indepth planning in consultation with experts in the field.

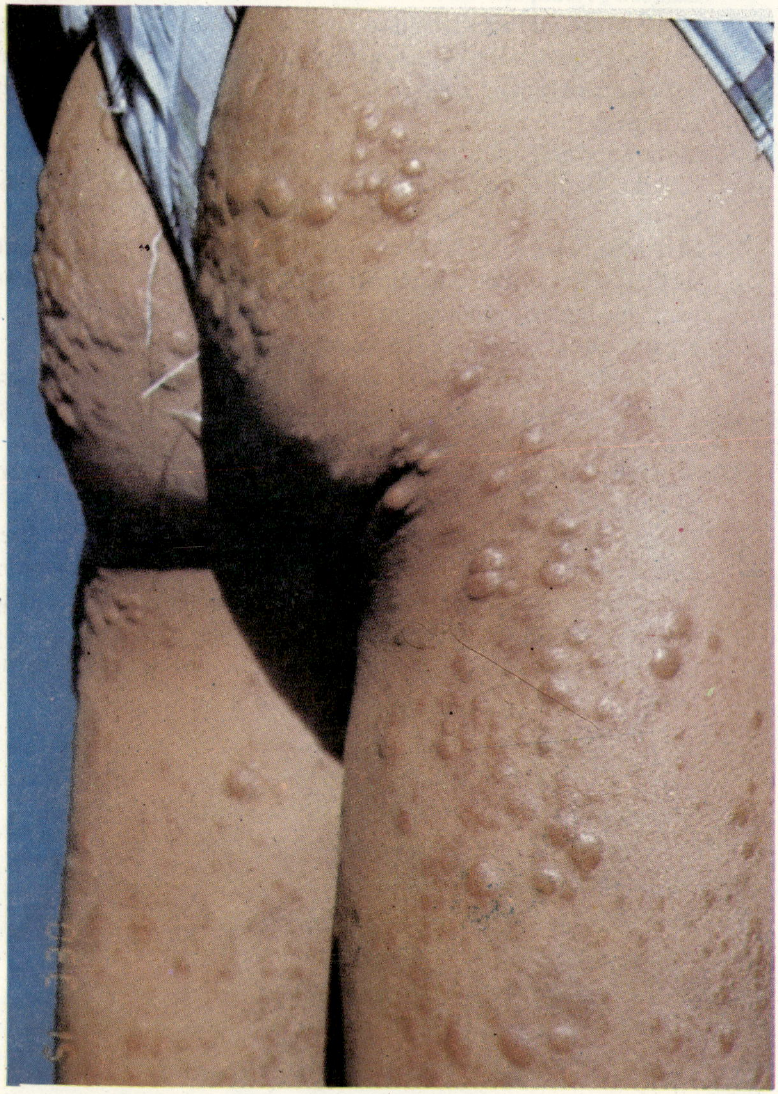

FIG. 7.1.1: Histoid Leprosy : LTC, Boko

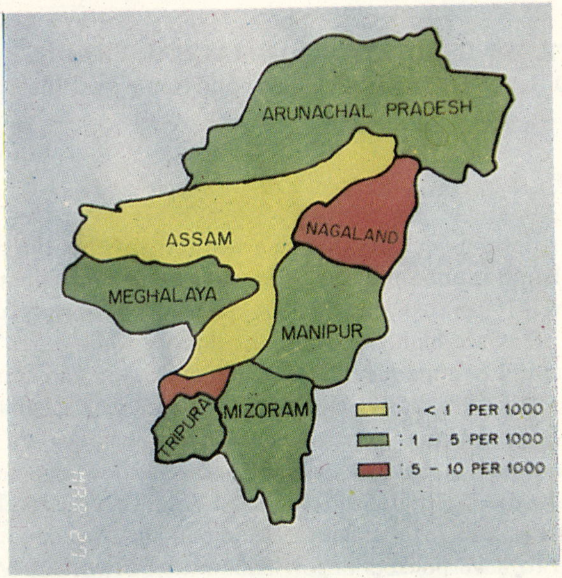

FIG. 7.1.2: Prevalence of Leprosy in N.E. States : Before MDT

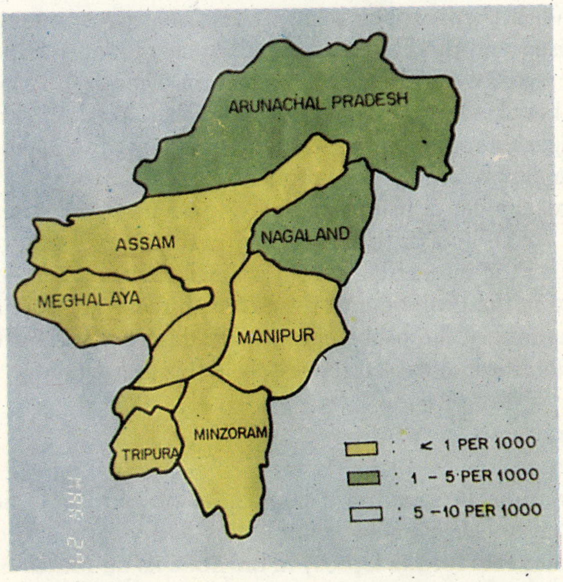

FIG. 7.1.3: Prevalence of Leprosy in N.E. States : After MDT, 1991

7.2 LEPROSY IN HARYAÑA, HIMACHAL PRADESH, PUNJAB AND CHANDIGARH: Problems and Some Possible Solutions

KIRAN KATOCH

India is a developing country with a vast territory but the distribution of population is not uniform – some area being more populated than other areas. Leprosy patients are also not uniformly distributed. Several areas are highly endemic for leprosy while other areas have moderate to low endemicity. Assam, Goa, Daman and Diu, Haryana, Himachal Pradesh, J&K, Meghalaya, Mizoram, Rajasthan, Tripura (all States) and Union Territories of Chandigarh, Dadara and Nagar Haveli and Delhi have been categorised as low endemic regions (Misra, 1990). The States of Arunachal Pradesh, Gujarat, Karnataka, Madhya Pradesh, Maharashtra, Manipur and Nagaland have been reported to have pockets of low endemicity. However, within these States also, there are pockets of varying endemicity in different districts. There is an increased awareness and determination to treat and eradicate leprosy. To achieve these objectives, strategies need to be devised and modified depending upon ground realities. Being a member of IV Independent Evaluation Team (IET) of NLEP in December 1991 for Haryana, Himachal Pradesh, Punjab and Chandigarh gave me an opportunity of gaining first hand experience of the magnitude of leprosy problem, its dynamics and efforts being made to combat it in this region. Apart from the statistical angle (Table 7.2.1), I plan to discuss my perceptions based on personal experience of interacting with technical and administrative people involved in the programme. Even though these are adjoining States, the dynamics of the problem are quite different and for this reason, these States are discussed separately in this presentation.

Haryana

The State of Haryana has a population of 1,63,17,715 according to 1991 Census, distributed in the cities and villages. The estimated prevalence rate for the leprosy in the State as on March 31, 1991 was 0.047/1000 population. There were a total of 780 recorded active cases (367 MB and 413 PB) in the State. Even though there is no vertical NLEP programme, these cases are on regular Multi-drug Therapy (MDT). Only 33 per cent of these cases are believed to be indigenous and 20-25 per cent of towns/cities and 2.5 per cent of villages seem to have the leprosy problem. Major part of the anti-leprosy programme in Haryana is being managed by the staff working in Tuberculosis Control Programme. Four Survey, Education and Training (SET) centres have been set up and three MDT districts have been sanctioned. Till October 1991, 140 general duty medical officers and 169 para-medical workers have been provided short-term orientation training in leprosy. Vehicles (2 sanctioned for leprosy) and microscopes are being used from the tuberculosis programme.

TABLE 7.2.1: Leprosy Situation in Northern States as on March 31, 1991

	Haryana	Himachal Pradesh	Punjab	Chandigarh
Prevalence rates	0.047/1000	0.77/1000	0.16/1000	2.8/1000
MB/PB cases	367-413	1973/1983	443/943	1059/984
Distribution	39/164 (cities) 158/6745 (villages)	Widely distributed	61/134 (cities) 327/12342 (villages)	—
Indigenous cases	33%	Origin not exactly known	30%	20-30%[1]
Treatment	MDT in Rohtak[2]	Monotherapy MDT in Solan District	MDT	MDT
Surveys	Active surveys started	SETs established; large trained infrastructure exists; no proper surveys conducted.	Sample surveys-cum-asssessment unit	Self reporting No surveys No staff

1. Old figures.
2. MDT in Karnal and Faridabad started later.

The districts of Sonepat and Ambala were reviewed by IV IET.

The district of Sonepat has a population of 7.4 lakhs with a prevalence rate of 0.047/1000. There is no separate staff and vehicle, provided for NLEP in the district and the programme, is being run by the Tuberculosis Control Programme. District Tuberculosis Officer (DTO) has been asked to look after the activities of NLEP in addition to his/her own duties. There were 13 recorded leprosy cases in the district, out of which 6 are MB and 7 PB — all of whom are on MDT. At present none of them are smear positive. No post of Zonal Leprosy Officer (ZLO), District Leprosy Officer (DLO), Medical Officer (MO), Non-Medical Supervisor (NMS), Para-Medical Worker (PMW), Health Educator (HE), Laboratory Technician, Physiotherapist, Smear Technician and Statistician has been sanctioned or provided for this or adjoining districts. Even as per State government figures, the supervisors, PMWs, AWNs and doctors serving in Sonepat, have not been provided any short or long term training for detection and treatment of leprosy cases. There is a post of MO for school children (such posts are there for other districts also) but the MO has not been provided any training or orientation course on leprosy. Inspite of the MO carrying out school surveys regularly, no proven or suspected case of leprosy has been detected. There is no microscope available and smears have to be sent to the district hospital for examination and reporting. The district has adequate stock of drugs for the NLEP activities. The staff of the PHC including the MO, MPW, HE needs to be trained to detect and diagnose early cases of leprosy.

The NLEP activities in the district of Ambala are being looked after by DLO. The total population is 11.06.275 and the prevalence rate has been estimated as 0.029/1000. On record, there are 32 leprosy cases in the district out of which 22 are MB and 10 are PB, all of them are under MDT. There is no post of MO, NMS, PMW, HE, Laboratory Technician, Physiotherapist, Smear Technician and Statistician in the NLEP programme. However, a general duty MO, who has been trained for 3 months in leprosy, carries out the anti-leprosy work in the district with the help of a skin specialist. There is no vehicle, microscope and laboratory equipment under the NLEP. The vehicle and microscope as also the service's of smear Technician of District Tuberculosis programme are being utilised for NLEP. There is adequate stock of drugs and the staff of the Ambala district hospital were found to be well oriented about the disease. They seemed to know each patient and his family members by name, and the community also had faith in them. The MPW also had imparted health education about leprosy to the community. The patients are taking their treatment regularly and records have been maintained satisfactorily. Here again the number of new MB patients detected have been higher than PB cases. There is facility for admission of leprosy patients at the district hospital. The DLO has been able to win the confidence of the local community and that of the medical and paramedical staff which has helped in implementing the NLEP without extra expenditure and staff. However, some more MOs and MPWs need re-orientation courses in leprosy to carry out the work more effectively.

Impressions

From the data provided by the State Government and personal experience of visiting the districts of Sonepat and Ambala, following impressions emerge:

(a) Even though there is no vertical programme, the problem seems to have been well tackled by the doctors and paramedical staff of general health care system, in this case by Tuberculosis Control personnel.

(b) Migrant population, in-coming due to economic reasons, seem to be contributing for more than 2/3 of the problem in the state. Such population needs special attention. It may be wiser to focus on the training of MOs and paramedical staff of Employees' State Insurance (ESI) dispensaries of the industrial units or closer to those areas where these populations are located.

(c) Although, on the basis of data available, one cannot draw confident conclusions about prevalence rates, etc., yet the problem seems to be localised to small number of villages and some towns. (Table 7.2.1). The health personnel in these areas should receive priority in getting the training. Similarly the MO, deployed for surveys, should also receive priority for these training programmes.

(d) In the document provided by the Haryana Government, emphasis on 'segregation' of cases have been laid. On checking, this was found not to be the policy, yet this shows misconceptions and prejudices even among some of the medical personnel. This may be reflecting just the social perceptions which are evident by the major portion of the cases being confined to the colonies. A massive effort to train medical and other personnel has been launched in Haryana. It is expected that, with the proper training of medical personnel about the disease, such misconceptions and prejudices will gradually go.

(e) NLEP consultants could help in monitoring the NLEP activities by undertaking small sample surveys from time to time as correct data about disease indices, like child case rate, deformity rates, etc., will be required in the future.

Chandigarh

All the data available about leprosy in Union Territory (UT) of Chandigarh is based on voluntary reporting. As on March 31, 1991, the prevalence of 2.8/1000 has been recorded in Chandigarh. At present there does not seem to be effective co-ordination between PGI which treats bulk of these cases and local health functionaries of UT and thus the data seems to be sketchy and may not be correct. 20-30 per cent of these cases are presumed to be indigenous. All the recorded cases – 1059 MB and 984 PB – in Chandigarh, are on MDT. Again, the major part of problem seems to be because of migrant population, and like Haryana it might be more profitable to provide training to general health care personnel giving priority to those who are located near the foci of these cases. Though the PGI may continue to serve as a referral centre, doctors and other personnel of dispensaries should be well trained and equipped to diagnose, treat and later on follow these cases. One Survey, Education and Treatment (SET) and one Urban Leprosy Centre (ULC) has been sanctioned for Chandigarh but due to want of recruitment rules, staff has not been recruited. Goitre cell staff of Chandigarh administration has been attending to leprosy, and facilities of the general hospital are being used for this programme.

Interestingly, like Haryana, all the status reports use the word "Leper" which again may be indicating a stigma in the minds of some of the medical people involved in the programme. Highlighting this terminology of 'Leper' or 'Segregation' by some odd medical doctors does not mean aspersions on overall picture in these areas or on committed medical and paramedical staff. But this is a reminder that prejudices even among some of the qualified people persist. It is hoped that the proper training of medical and other categories of general health service will help in reducing this stigma. After a network of these services becomes available, proper channels to collect all the data should be developed.

Punjab

The data presented to IET team shows a prevalence rate of 0.16/1000 population in Punjab. As on March 31, 1991, there were 443 MB and 943 PB recorded cases of leprosy. Like Haryana and Chandigarh, 20-30 per cent of leprosy cases are believed to be indigenous; remaining are migrant people from other States. These cases have been reported from half of the towns/cities, only from 2-5 per cent of villages, and nearly 50 per cent of them are living in the leprosy colonies. There are 12 Urban Leprosy Centres (ULCs) working under the supervision of DLO with one urban leprosy worker. Four upgraded urban leprosy centers are being supervised by MOs, all of them being skin specialists. All the diagnosed cases are being treated with MDT. Except for 5 NMSs and some PMWs, all other posts under NLEP have been filled up by qualified and well trained staff (7 MOs, one senior PMWs, 8 PMW and 4 Laboratory Technicians) and there seems to be concerted efforts to provide training to general health cadre medical doctors and other categories of the staff. Other infra-structure facilities, such as vehicles, microscopes and health education material are available. The fact that most of the MOs working in the programme are skin specialists, appears to be good and proper deployment of qualified manpower. Further, like Ambala in Haryana, the paramedical staff of general health care like MPWs were found to be well motivated and in good rapport with community in these areas (Mohali and Ropar were evaluated by IET). Even still better results can be expected by properly rewarding these personnel.

Sample Survey-cum-Assessment Unit established in 1987-88 under the NLEP programme has started functioning. Although NMS, PMW and Smear Technician for the unit have not been recruited, the unit has detected new cases including child cases from 'suspect' populations. The approach needs to be strengthened in neighbouring states of Haryana, Himachal Pradesh and Chandigarh as well. Seeing the trends and efforts being made in training of medical and other categories of personnel, Punjab should be able to effectively tackle the problem and hopefully leprosy colonies would become a thing of the past. The migrant population and other areas showing the foci of infection should receive the priority, as suggested for Haryana and Chandigarh also.

Himachal Pradesh

As on March 31, 1991, Himachal Pradesh had 3956 registered cases of leprosy and overall estimated prevalence rate was 0.77/1000. Leprosy cases have been reported from almost all the districts with prevalence rates ranging from 0.03 to 1.88/1000. Overall MB/PB ratio is almost 1:1 The programme is being run through 6 Leprosy Control Units (LCUs), 79 peripheral clinics and 15 SET centres. There are 14 Assistant Leprosy Officers and 64 leprosy workers (34 trained) recruited for NLEP. In addition, there is a ULC with Medical College, Shimla, a Reconstructive Surgical Unit and 232 indoor beds for leprosy patients. Dapsone monotherapy is still practised all over the State (except for Solan district).

IET had the opportunity of touring Sirmaur and Solan districts and the impressions are discussed in the following paragraphs.

The district headquarters of Sirmaur are situated at Nahan. The population of this district is 3,78,800 with a prevalence rate of 1.88 per 1000. The river Giri divides this district into two regions, the Trans-Giri (beyond the Giri river) and Cis-Giri track. The whole area is divided into 15 leprosy sub-units with higher endemicity in Trans-Giri areas. There is one post of MO and two posts of Assistant Leprosy Officers which are filled-up in the district. Dapsone monotherapy is being given in the district. Overall nine posts of leprosy workers have been filled-up against 15 sanctioned posts. Most of the leprosy workers and MOs have been trained. One vehicle is available, but it is considered inadequate because of scattered population and difficult terrain of district. The distance from one village to another varies from 3 to 10 km and in the Trans-Giri area the roads are not motorable in many areas. There is a temporary hospitalization ward with one nurse posted there. The hospitalised patients get MDT. Some of the leprosy workers are well trained and have gained the confidence of the community, while others are not so well motivated to perform their duties. There is a Laboratory Technician with microscope and necessary reagents. The stock of drugs is also adequate. The MB rate is 41 per cent in the newly diagnosed cases of leprosy. The purpose of discussing these details is to highlight the fact, that infrastructure to launch the MDT programme exists. Because of slow response to Dapsone monotherapy, the NLEP is not popular. Although the terrain is difficult, with a little training to general care paramedical and medical staff, MDT can be implemented as it has been done in Haryana.

The Zonal Leprosy Officer is stationed at Solan. This area has a population of 3,30,000 scattered in an area of 1936 sq km with a prevalence rate of 0.36 per 1000. The 75 bedded leprosy hospital is situated at Mandodhar which has a MO, one Assistant Leprosy Officer, 2 staff nurses, 3 pharmacists, 2 Laboratory Technicians and 4 leprosy workers at its staff. Among them, one leprosy worker was not trained. These are 192 cases of leprosy in this district, out of which 113 are MB and 79 PB. All of them were on regular MDT. Among the new cases detected, the ratio of MB to PB cases is 2:1. The staff is trained but, as allowance for leprosy workers is not given as in endemic districts, most of the leprosy workers do not go to the field and work enthusiastically for NLEP. The State Leprosy Officer (SLO) and MO have pooled in the resources of the voluntary agencies, like Rotary Club which is trying to help in rehabilitation of leprosy patients. The vehicle for NLEP is out of order and is not repairable. A vehicle is urgently required considering the location of villages and difficult terrain. The general health care workers are not sufficiently aware of the disease and trained, and consequently the community is also not aware of the disease and of newer effective treatment. The Para-medical staff insists on special allowance for working in leprosy as is being given to the leprosy workers of verticle programme. More Primary Health Care workers should be trained and motivated to work in leprosy. MDT should be started in all the districts of Himachal Pradesh as it has been done in Haryana and Punjab. There is adequate basic health staff and it should be motivated and mobilised to work for NLEP.

Overall, the magnitude of the problem seems to be much more in Himachal Pradesh as compared to neighbouring States. Also, the leprosy cases appear to be widely scattered unlike the neighbouring States where migrant populations seem to be important foci and can be concentrated upon. Introduction of the MDT all over the State, training and motivation of medical and other categories of personnel, provision of sufficient vehicles for field visits, review of policy of giving leprosy allowance are important measures which need to be taken up in Himachal Pradesh to strengthen the leprosy programme. Himachal Pradesh has an excellent network of public health services and these can be geared up to diagnose and treat leprosy.

Conclusion

As discussed in the preceding paragraphs, Haryana, Himachal Pradesh, Punjab and Chandigarh continue to be endemic for leprosy. The rates of MB : PB cases is around 1:1, thus conforming to intermediary phase of epidemiology of leprosy (Misra, et al, 1989; WHO, 1985). An overview of recent literature shows that position has not changed dramatically in the recent past (Dharmshaktu, et al, 1987; Kant, 1990; Kaul, et al, 1982; Misra, et al, 1989; Misra, 1990; Singh, 1990). Some aspects like migrant populations, difficulty in reaching the areas, etc., would be peculiar to some of these states and regions, but most of other problems are common. For example –

(a) The small magnitude of the problem in these low endemic States does not require a vertical programme. In fact, the success of personnel working in general health care and other programmes in Haryana and Punjab shows that integrated approach can work very well.
(b) Orientation and training of MOs and, wherever available, proper deployment of specialists and trained manpower is necessary for diagnosing and treating the leprosy early, scientifically and without prejudice/fear. The training of various categories of workers including MPWs, Laboratory Technicians (Rao, et al, 1987) needs special attention.
(c) The practice of giving leprosy allowance, etc., should be seriously reviewed as this seems to be counter-productive and may turn out to be a major stumbling block in the integration and effective participation of general health care system in the NLEP. This issue needs urgent attention as implementation of modified MDT in moderately endemic districts (DGHS, 1990) and MDT in low endemic areas, which has already been proposed in some areas (Mukherjee, 1990), will depend largely upon the morale and active participation of general health care staff.
(d) As suggested by Misra and Sharma, a network of peripheral and

referral facilitie to provide the services for treatment of leprosy should be provided (Misra, 1990; Sharma, 1990). Such system will also help in gaining meaningful statistical data about indices, like child leprosy rates, disability rates, relapses and reaction after MDT, etc., which are vital for monitoring the success of the programme. At present, there is no worthwhile data about these indices at least in the above States.

(e) Sample survey teams should be established in all these States and, after planning a well-coordinated strategy, sample surveys should be immediately carried out.

(f) Extension of MDT to several low endemic areas has already been proposed (Mukherjee, 1990). But this is not enough and MDT should be given to all the patients in all low endemic areas. We need not wait till the low endemic areas turn into high endemic zones (Bedi, 1990). As the optimum duration for current MDT is still being debated, an integral network of services for obtaining feedback during and after the MDT should be made available.

It needs to be emphasized that the battle in the low endemic areas will be a long one and that it would require dynamic changes in the strategies from time to time. Lessons from recent past pinpoint certain areas and foci to concentrate upon in these States. Our efforts in this presentation would serve the purpose if it succeeds in focussing on these issues so as to get maximum benefit from recent advances achieved in improving the treatment of leprosy.

REFERENCES

Bedi, B.M.S., 1990, Monitoring of MDT in Endemic and Low-endemic Areas, *in, Report of Workshop on MDT of Low-endemic Areas: An Evaluation*, Safdarjang Hospital, New Delhi, p 74-76.

Dharmshaktu, N.S.; Sharma, R.C.; Devarajan, L.; Mittal, B.N., 1987, A Survey on Proportion of Multibacillary Cases of Leprosy in Himachal Pradesh, *Indian J. Lepr*, 59, p 300-308.

Kant, R., 1990, District Jalandhar, Punjab, Status Report, *in, Report of Workshop on MDT of Low-endemic Areas: An Evaluation*, Safdarjang Hospital, New Delhi, p 85-86.

Kaul, S.; Kumar, B.; Roy, S.N., 1982, Endemicity of Leprosy in the Union Territory of Chandigarh and Surrounding States, *Lepr India*, 54, p 428-440.

Misra R.S., 1990, Strategy for Leprosy Eradication Programme in Low-endemic Areas, *in, Report of Workshop on MDT of Low-endemic Areas: An Evaluation*, Safdarjang Hospital, New Delhi, p 23-32.

Misra, R.S.; Ramesh, V.; Nigam, P.K., 1989, Leprosy in Low-endemic Areas of India: An Appraisal and Suggested Measures for Control, *Indian J Lepr*, 61, p 345-350.

Mukherjee, A.K., 1990, Inaugural Address, *in, Report of Workshop on MDT of Low-endemic Areas: An Evaluation*, Safdarjang Hospital, New Delhi, p 13-15.

NLEP, 1990, *Guidelines for Modified MDT Scheme in Selected Districts, National Leprosy Eradication in India*, Leprosy Division, Directorate General of Health Services, New Delhi.

Rao, C.K.; Dharmshaktu, N.S.; Mittal, B.N.; Roychaudhary, S.B.; Shah, N.K.; Kumar, S., 1987, National Leprosy Eradication Programme in India. An Independent Evaluation, *Indian J Lepr*, 59, p 203-218.

Sharma, N.K., 1990, Role of Specialised Centres in Leprosy Control Programme, *in, Report of Workshop on MDT of Low-endemic Areas: An Evaluation*, Safdarjang Hospital, New Delhi, p 77-80.

Singh, R.M., 1990, Bighupur District, Manipur: Status Report, *in, Report of Workshop on MDT of Low-endemic Areas: An Evaluation,* Safdarjang Hospital, New Delhi, p 88-90.

WHO, 1985, *WHO Technical Report Series,* WHO Study Group, Geneva, Switzerland, No. 716, p 43.

7.3 LEPROSY ERADICATION IN RAJASTHAN AND JAMMU REGION (J&K STATE)

R.S. MISRA

Pream

The observations recorded in this chapter are based on the findings of the IV Independent Evaluation of National Leprosy Eradication Programme, December, 12-20, 1991, by the joint Government of India – World Health Organisation Team, consisting of:

Team Leader
Dr. V. Ekambram, President, Indian Association of Leprologists, Madras.

Members
Dr. Anand Raj, National Leprosy Consultant
Dr. C. McDougall, International Expert (U.K.)

Member Secretary
Dr. R.S. Misra

Rajasthan

The State of Rajasthan covers a geographical area of 342267 sq km, approximating around 10 per cent of the total land area of the country. This land mass can mainly be categorised into (a) deserts of erstwhile Marwad, (b) fertile plains with cities of Alwar, Bharatpur, Jaipur, Sawai Madhopur, etc., and (c) Hilly tribal belt, covering the districts of Udaipur, Chittorgarh, Banswara, Dungarpur, Sirohi and Bundi. The total population of the State, as per 1991 Census is 4,38,80,640, registering an increase of 25 per cent over the last 1981 Census figures, with a density of population of 1281 sq km.

A total of 23,032 leprosy cases were recorded by March 1991, against an estimated case-load of 10,000. Thirteen districts have a prevalence of 2-3.5/1000. Thirteen districts have a prevalence of 2-3.5/1000 and the remaining less than 2/1000 population (Table

7.3.1). In six out of 27 districts the programme is operated under NLEP.

TABLE 7.3.1: Districtwise Number of Cases Detected and Discharged alongwith Prevalence Rate up to March 1991

Sl. No.	District	Cases Detected up to March, 1991	Type of cases Detected		No. of cases Discharged		Total Cases Dis-charged	Preva-lence Rate
			M.B.	P.B.	M.B.	P.B.		
01.	Alwar	2017	703	1314	455	868	1323	2.23
02.	Ajmer	853	286	567	136	236	372	2.83
03.	Banswara	614	205	409	49	100	149	2.08
04.	Bharatpur	2247	740	1507	172	305	477	3.11
05.	Bhilwara	79	26	53	—	—	—	—
06.	Bikaner	675	227	448	34	68	102	1.86
07.	Bundi	248	83	165	18	37	55	2.60
08.	Chittorgarh	252	84	168	23	48	71	1.98
09.	Churu	146	48	98	10	21	31	1.05
10.	Dholpur	471	157	314	86	172	258	2.73
11.	Dungarpur	525	175	350	34	68	102	2.19
12.	Ganganagar	153	51	102	1	3	4	2.66
13.	Jaipur	5560	1892	3668	477	850	1327	1.36
14.	Jaisalmer	75	25	50	11	21	32	1.35
15.	Jhalawar	317	105	212	17	35	52	
16.	Jhunjhunu	618	206	412	68	137	205	1.33
17.	Jodhpur	1524	517	1007	244	490	734	1.34
18.	Kota	534	178	356	68	138	206	1.90
19.	Nagaur	3118	1046	2072	587	1105	1692	1.79
20.	Pali	193	64	129	14	28	42	2.53
21.	Sawai Madhopur	508	169	339	34	69	103	3.56
22.	Sikar	463	154	309	49	101	150	2.85
23.	Sirohi	162	54	108	13	28	41	3.51
24.	Tonk	39	13	26	10	20	30	—
25.	Udaipur	1632	558	1074	43	65	108	2.71
	Total	23023	7766	15257	2653	5013	7666	2.25

The Independent Evaluation Team (IET) visited three districts of Alwar, Jaipur and Bharatpur out of the six districts in which NLEP is in operation. The performance of the Centre in the area was assessed qualitatively as well as quantitatively on the basis of available facts and figures and interviewing and interacting with health-personnel in the programme from State Leprosy Officer (SLO), District Leprosy

Officers (DLOs), Medical Officers (MOs), down to Para-medical Workers (PMWs), Non-medical Supervisors (NMSs), Laboratory Technicians, patients, the community leaders and contacts of the patients in the family and village, etc.

Relevant Observations

(1) The case-detection has not gone on as actively as desired due to various difficulties of logistics.

(2) A large number of posts of PMWs remain unfilled. Even all those in position are not trained, on an average, at least 50 per cent require immediate training to be utilised gainfully in the control programme. Even the trained PMWs need refresher courses of training to make them conversant with the latest changes in the operative strategies.

(3) Due to difficult field conditions and the lack of transport at their disposal and restricted tour days sanctioned by the State Government the supervisory medical personnel, namely, SLO, DLOs and MOs and MOs of Leprosy Control Units (LCUs) have been unable to exercise the necessary supervision and guidance.

(4) Temporary Hospitalisation Ward (THW) in existence and built with great foresight at Deeg has remained unutilised due to financial constraints and lack of managerial promptness on the part of the State.

(5) *Role of Voluntary Agencies* – Non-governmental Organisations (NGOs) and voluntary agencies can perform the important role of coordinating the social effort with medical facilities. In this respect many voluntary agencies, like Damien Foundation, Sarthak Manav Kusht Ashram (Jaipur), Bhagwan Mahaveer Sahayata Kushta Sewa Samiti, etc., are doing good work in the State. The team visited Sarthak Manav Kusht Ashram, Jaipur, where it found that the clinical and rehabilitative aspects of leprosy patients and their families are being looked after. A commendable effort is also made to provide Micro Cellular Rubber (MCR) shoes/chappals to any patient of leprosy from the State or outside free of cost.

(6) The whole-effort of Leprosy Eradication needs a coordinated and cohesive working to make it successful in the short span of time in future.

Jammu Region (J&K State)

The whole State of Jammu and Kashmir (J&K) is divided into three regions, namely, (i) Kashmir Valley, (ii) Ladakh, and (iii) Jammu. The Jammu region has an area of 26239 sq km with a population of 30.3 Lakhs (1991 Census) spread over 6 districts in the region. The terrain is hilly with a sparse population density of 115/sq km. The population is mainly dependent on agriculture and not economically well off. The literacy rate is only 27 per cent.

The State is categorised as low-endemic for leprosy. A survey conducted by Late Dr. Dharmendra in 1965 for the whole State of J&K recorded a prevalence of 5/1000 population with an estimated 20,000 cases. As per latest records 3702 leprosy cases (MB 1030, PB 2672) have been detected and brought under regular treatment.

NLEP was launched in the State in 1963. So far 6 LCUs, 15 SET Centres and the Urban Leprosy Centre (ULC) have been established. MDT was introduced in 1987-88 in Jammu region on the initiative of the State Government itself. At present 730 cases (522 MB and 208 PB) are under MDT. So far 2972 cases have been released from treatment after MDT and are under surveillance.

The team visited LCUs and PHCs in the Kathua and Udhampur districts, interviewed NLEP as well as PHC staff, patients, community leaders and its members. The team also visited the patients at their homes and verified the diagnosis and survey work. The implementation of the programme was discussed with CMOs, Health and Family Welfare of the districts, Professor of Dermatology and Vernereology at State Government Medical College at Jammu, Director of Health and Medical Services and Secretary (Health) of the State.

Observations

1. The progress of the NLEP is much hampered because of:

   (a) Lack of updated knowledge of leprosy in the programme implementation staff, viz., MOs, MPWs of PHCs.
   (b) Untrained NLEP staff, e.g., MOs of LCUs and PMWs.
   (c) Lack of re-training for those, who had their training long years back and are in need of updating their knowledge.

2. The health-education is very inadequate and is thus not having the desired effect on reducing the stigma in the community or in encouraging voluntary reporting of leprosy cases.
3. The mobility of NLEP staff is curtailed due to non-availability of the vehicle to the MOs of LCUs and other supervisory staff.
4. About 2000 patients with anaesthetic feet requiring footwears are identified but there is no provision for the supply of footwears.
5. In the ULC attached to the Government Medical College, Jammu, 1399 cases are registered but only less than half have completed the schedule of treatment because of physical difficulties in attending the Centre from far-off areas of the State. This calls for a closer liaison between NLEP staff and ULC at Medical College, to guarantee the complete supervised treatment of diagnosed cases.
6. There are no facilities in the State for training of the Programme personnel.

Recommendations for Improving the Working of LEP

1. The observations made with regard to the above two low-endemic states of the country has brought to fore the most important point that no recent factual assessment of the quantum of the problem is available. This calls for immediate sample surveys in such low-endemic areas to correctly quantitate the problem.
2. All efforts in NLEP should be geared towards the early diagnosis, and full and regular treatment, as per guidelines of NLEP. It has been the experience of all the workers in these low-endemic areas that due to various factors, viz., lack of health-education, economic difficulties, etc., the failure of regular treatment is the most important impediment in the eradication of disease. For this, the linkages among (i) leprosy diagnostician, be he at LCU, ULC or SET Centre or be he a private practitioner of Dermatology and Leprology/Professor in a Medical College, (ii) personnel of Primary Health Centre/Sub-Centre in the area of vicinity of the leprosy patient, and (iii) village community level leader/worker, are to be strengthened. All these three will have to work in complete unison to ensure a regular treatment for leprosy patients,

because in almost 85 per cent cases, the patient does not face reactions and other complications following the start of treatment.

3. But, for approximately 20 per cent cases of leprosy, where the patient may face 'exacerbations' in the disease following start of anti-leprosy treatment, disabilities due to antecedent disease, by way of anaesthetic feet and hands, etc., should be carefully looked into and sympathetically explained. For example, the anaesthetic hands and feet, which may be a matter of fact result of the disease for the clinician and PMWs, can be a cause of great concern to the leprosy patient. This needs to be explained in detail taking into account the common precautions which ought to be observed by the patient to prevent the deformities and disabilities following the anaesthetic limbs. Severe reactions and disabilities should be handled by admitting the patient to THW or undertaking reconstructive surgery at appropriate centre.
4. The NLEP, following introduction of MDT, has mainly concentrated on ensuring the complete treatment and on making the patient non-infective over a stipulated period of time, without taking full care of non-infective patients with anaesthetic hands and feet and without ensuring them or advising them non-hurting proper foot-wears and suitable appliances to protect their anaesthetic hands at work or in the absence of it alternate vocational training.
5. The personnel, engaged in leprosy eradication work or likely to participate in it following integration of NLEP with PHC set-up, should receive adequate training in advance to be able to cope up with the handling of leprosy patients with their updated knowledge on the subject. Under the programme, the DLOs, MOs, etc., should have sufficient mobility and be provided vehicle exclusively meant for the programme. This should also be supported by frequent exchange of information among all levels of personnel and feedback on the activities of the programme in the area under their control in order to take corrective steps in time.
6. Health education is one of the most important inputs which is to be introduced with full thought and foresight, and taking into account the local socio-cultural milieu and regional peculiarities. One thing considered good at one place may not

be universally acceptable. The health-education activities are to be further assessed in the context of Knowledge-Attitude-Practices (KAP) and for it the social-scientists have to constantly evaluate the content of the health-education material. The various media, e.g., press, radio, TV, film, skits, fares, etc., are to be exploited, as per local suitability and susceptibility.

7. Voluntary Agencies and NGOs in many areas are doing yeoman's service. The Voluntary Agencies imported from outside can help only to a certain degree, and that too if, by their humanitarian work, they have been able to touch the human chord in the local populace. Thus these agencies can help the community in changing their attitudes and prejudicial social practices against the leprosy afflicted individuals. But, the ideal will be, for the community leaders at various levels, say, village, *mohalla* or block to come forward and enthuse the local people to organise into such voluntary groups and help in their limited way by acting as an ideal link between the medical personnel-patient-society on either side, so that the regularity of treatment without default or irregularity and social acceptance of the patient without losing his/her dignity and social status, by way of his/her occupation or job and in the instance of his/her disability to continue in his/her present job due to his/her deformity or injuriousness to his/her limbs. This should not be allowed to happen due to social rejection. By providing him/her with an alternate job/occupation, or training for the new one, the society can help the patient in sustaining him/her in a crucial phase. This will help him/her not only in maintaining his/her dignity and income, but will stop the process of dehabilitation and strengthening of the stigma against the disease.

PART IV

PROBLEMS IN LEPROSY MANAGEMENT

8

PROGRESSION OF DISEASE AND REACTIONS IN LEPROSY

G. RAMU

It is expedient to consider worsening of the disease and methods of assessing the effect of therapy before differentiating it from reaction. It will not be out of place to consider the essential features of reactions in order to have a clear concept of the two clinical entities.

Factors Leading to Mistakes in Diagnosis of Progression

1. The worsening may be more apparent than real. A lot of expectation has been generated about the efficacy of Multi-drug Therapy (MDT) both among the lay public and the workers about the cure of the disease. When borderline lesions subside they leave behind in some individuals marked hypopigmentation which might not have been so noticeable when the lesions were coppery coloured on a dark skin. The conspicuous hypopigmentation is often interpreted as worsening. The workers also tend to believe that there is extension of the disease.
2. A real progression is seen among cases when there is premature termination of treatment due to mistakes in categorisation of patients as Pauci-bacillary (PB) when the patient had Multi-bacillary (MB) leprosy.
3. Difficulty arises in assessing the activity of flat or macular lesions where two important signs, the subsidence of which helps in diagnosing activity are absent from the beginning. They are, (a) erythema, and (b) infiltration or thickening.
4. A few cases, where treatment is stopped before the commencement of regression, become worse.

To guard against these mistakes some clinical methods are suggested.

Modification in Assessing Clinical Progress in PB Leprosy

In PB leprosy (Tuberculoid and Indeterminate) with one to three lesions, it will be useful to measure the lesions in two directions at points of maximum length. This could be entered in the chart depicting the lesions. In macular lesions there should not be (i) any increase in the extent of the lesion, and/or (ii) the appearance of new lesions at the time of releasing from treatment. In infiltrated lesions this will be useful and it will be reassuring to know that there is no increase in the size.

Assessment of Lesions of Borderline Leprosy

Borderline leprosy encompasses a spectrum of lesions with different morphological characteristics which varies between individual patients and in the same patient at different times. An objective rating of the number and extent of lesions is considered in borderline leprosy. Either several lesions varying in size from small, i.e., less than two cm to five cm or extensive lesions covering large part of a sector may be found. For assessment of number, the body is divided into seven sectors, namely, (1) Head and neck, (2) Right upper limb, (3) Left upper limb, (4) Trunk, (5) Gluteal region and genitalia, (6) Right lower limb, and (7) Left lower limb.

If the lesions are small or medium, i.e., less than five cm when measured in either of two directions, the number of lesions are taken into account and given numerical scores in each sectors as given in Table 8.1.

TABLE 8.1: Number of Lesions and Their Score

Sl. No.	Number of Lesions	Score
1.	None	0
2.	1-3	1
3.	4-5	2
4.	6-9	3
5.	10 and over	4

The lesions scattered in different parts of the body and earning a score of nine or within nine are considered to form PB leprosy. Trunk-nerve involvement is considered a lesion. When the score is over three, i.e., the number of lesions is above nine, the disease is categorised as MB for purposes of treatment.

If during assessment the clinical score increases in the absence of a reactional state, it should be termed as worsening.

When lesions are extensive, i.e., more than five cm and occupying large areas they are given the score as given in Table 8.2 in comparison to the above.

TABLE 8.2: Percentage of Involvement: Its Score

Sl. No.	Extent of involvement in one sector	Score
1.	Up to 25%	1
2.	26-49%	2
3.	50-74%	3
4.	75% and above	4

Patients with a score of three in three sectors would be considered MB. If the score increases during assessment, the disease will be considered worsening.

In polyneuritic leprosy fresh nerve involvement would be considered to be worsening.

Rationale for Above Considerations

It is appropriate to point out that BT leprosy patients have been shown to have bacillaemia (Raval, et al, 1982). Antibody levels were found to be increased in tuberculoid patients having widespread form of the disease (Touw, et al, 1983). BT leprosy patients with multiple lesions were found to have increased antibody levels using SACT and PGL I ELISA (Kanchana, et al, n.d.). Nerves were shown to have bacilli even when the skin smears were negative (Arunthathi, 1988). It has been observed that cases with a larger number of nerves involved were fraught with more relapses (Grungi, et al, 1990; Ramu, et al, 1974; Chopra, et al, 1990; Ramu, et al, 1988).

Lesions extend by advancing at the periphery over a period of time and by the coalescing of satellite lesions. The extent of the lesions, therefore, suggests the presence of undetected organisms.

Torpid TT and BT Lesions

Occasionally lesions are encountered which do not regress in size, erythema or infiltration. Perhaps they represent primary resistant PB leprosy. They call for addition of clofazimine.

Assessment of Lepromatous Leprosy

A popular misconception that finds its way into guides for health workers is that MDT cures leprosy in a short time. While field reports on MB patients show a rapid bacteriological clearance, reports on drug trials of BL and lepromatous leprosy (Katoch, et al, 1989; Thomas, et al, 1990) indicate that very few become negative bacteriologically even after four years of regular therapy. On the basis of mouse foot-pad studies, however, it is observed that the bacilli become non-viable after a few doses. The BI falls at the rate of 0.6 to one log unit per year under MDT. There are, however, individual variations. A patient with BI of five at the beginning of treatment would have a BI of three or more after two years. This does not mean that the disease is refractory and resistance is to be suspected but instead the immunological response is tardy and does not clear the dead bacilli.

The significant observation is clinical improvement which sets in faster than bacteriological improvement. This was commensurate with a fall in MI in centres where expertise was available. For assessing clinical improvement a system of semi-quantitative numerical scoring has been in use at Central Leprosy Traning and Research Institute, Chinglepattu, (Iyer, et al, 1977), Central Jalme Institute of Leprosy, Agra, Tuberculosis Research Centre, Madri, and National Institute of Immunology, New Delhi, for assessing cases under different therapeutic regimens. The numerical scores are assigned to the various types of skin lesions in lepromatous leprosy initially and during periodic assessment. The body is divided into seven sectors as mentioned before. The clinical scores allotted to the different lesions are given in Table 8.3.

TABLE 8.3: Character of Lesions and Their Score

1.	Macules and fine infiltration manifesting as shiny	1
2.	Well marked infiltration with prominent skin markings	2
3.	Very thick infiltration with occasional papules or nodules	3
4.	Nodules, thick papules and plaques	4

The predominant lesion in the particular sector of the body is taken for scoring. The scores in the different regions are added up. Thus, in a given case if all the seven sectors have a score of four each, the total score will be 28. With improvement, papules, plaques, nodules and thick infiltration start regressing. The thick papules, plaques and nodules present a shrivelled appearance with an overlying thinned out skin. Nodules present pricked bubble appearance. Increase in clinical scores is due to increase in infiltration or appearance of papules and nodules afresh. This may occur during treatment if the therapy is inadequate or after release from therapy (RFT) when there is worsening. While, by and large, MDT is effective, in these days when, in some centres, treatment is terminated after a fixed duration of therapy for two years, it is advisable to chart patients with care and allot scores initially, periodically, at RFT and during surveillance. Increase in the score occurs ahead of bacteriological worsening.

Very often hypodermal or subcutaneous nodules may be the first manifestation of deterioration. In the beginning, they feel like peas in a pod both in size and consistency. Later they increase in size. The common sites are posterior and lateral aspects of arms, buttocks, thighs, dorsum of hands and lower part of back. These are subcutanceous histoids. Care should be taken to fix the nodules with two fingers, and plunge the point of the scalpel into the core of the nodule. Taking smears from the overlying skin will not be helpful. The bacilli would be plentiful, long and tapering and not as per description of Shepard and McRae (Ramanujam, et al, 1969).

Increase in infiltration occurs over the dorsum of hands, fingers and toes; papules and nodules appear over the inner side of the eyebrows, posterior aspect of arms, lower part of the back. One should also look into the nose, eyes, palate and the scrotum. Early papules and young nodules are pink in colour.

The Reactional States

Reactional states represent heightened immunologic responses to M. leprae or its breakdown products manifested as acute inflammation in the skin and/or nerve and/or other sites. As in the case of active leprosy, a spectrum can be observed in reactional states also. Reactions can be identified as BT, BB or BL. Tuberculoid reactions are very uncommon. For uniformity the term "reversal reaction" was recommended in the workshop sponsored by the Indian Association of Leprologists (IAL) and Government of India in 1986, avoiding a multiplicity of terms such as Type I and upgrading reaction. In lepromatous leprosy the reactions have been termed as "ENL Syndrome".

Frequency of Reactional States

In MB leprosy reversal reactions were encountered in 23 per cent and ENL in 13.5 per cent. In PB patients eight cases were seen out of 1050 patients.

The Time of Onset of Reactions

Eighty per cent of reversal reactions and 64 per cent of episodes of ENL syndrome occur in the first six months of therapy. This is earlier than the experience with dapsone where reactions occurred after nine months of therapy. Reversal reactions have been encountered for as long as two years and ENL for more than three years in those who experience recurring episodes. They averaged 2.8 for ENL syndrome and 1.7 for reversal reaction. While reversal reactions are seen mostly among those who were bacteriologically positive, a few are observed in those with negative smears. In such cases neuritis (acute painful neuritis) is seen, the reaction in the skin lesions being not very prominent.

The ENL syndrome encompasses a variety of skin and systemic manifestations besides constitutional disturbances. The skin manifestations include exacerbation of existing lesions, namely, macules, infiltration, plaques and nodules. An exacerbation may involve mucous membrane lesions as well. The new lesions in ENL syndrome consist of ENL, erythema multiforme and subcutaneous nodules. The systemic manifestations of ENL syndrome are neuritis, arthritis, anterior uveitis, myositis, orchitis, lymphadenitis, osteoperiostis, etc. (Table 8.4).

TABLE 8.4: Differences between ENL Syndrome and Relapsed Papules and Young Histoid

	ENL syndrome	Relapsed papules and young histoid
History of Therapy	During therapy and as episodes, in LL, LLs, rarely BL	During inadequate therapy, or after long interrupted therapy, or irregular therapy, BB, BL, LLs, LL.
Constitutional signs	Present	Absent
Physical Exam.	Redness, Tenderness, Warmth	Pink not tender not warm
	ENL are superficial.	Involve whole thickness of skin.
Course	Undergo colour changes becoming blue, then dark subsiding in 48-72 hours. Occur in crops and blanch on pressure. Exacerbation of existing lesions last for a week or more, and subside with desquamation. Rarely vesiculation, pustulation and ulceration may occur.	Long lasting. Pink colour gives place to skin colour with a firmer consistency.
Skin smears	Bleeding while taking smears. Smears reveal several PMN; highly fragmented AFB may be in PMN.	B.I. 3 or more, Long tapering, AFB in histoid (Ramanujan and Ramu, 1969)

The subcutaneous Histoid nodules have to be differentiated from the subcutaneous nodules which occur in recurrent attacks of ENL syndrome (Table 8.4). While subcutaneous Histoid occurs in inadequately treated patients of borderline or lepromatous leprosy, subcutaneous nodules arise in those patients under therapy who are subject to repeated reactive states. The lesions which were originally answering the description of ENL become deeper involving the entire skin, and later infiltrating the subcutaneous tissue and even the underlying structures. These nodules are tender unlike the subcutaneous histoid; they are attached to the overlying skin. The skin may be hyperpigmented if the attack of reaction has been recent. Skin smears present a large number of PMN with fragmented organisms.

While dealing with the subject of reaction in lepromatous leprosy, it is useful to point out that erythema multiforme lesions may sometimes masquerade as borderline leprosy lesions. Erythema multiforme lesions are of acute onset, accompanied by constitutional symptoms and appear as papular eruptions; they enlarge or more papular eruptions arise at the periphery and fuse creating a red blotch. The middle of the blotch changes in colour to blue, the peripheral part being red. Later this gives way to a dark hue and subsides with slight desquamation. This resembles the circinate lesions of borderline leprosy (BL). The distinguishing sign is the blanching of the red peripheral portion on pressure and tenderness besides the tell-tale history. Smears as in ENL reveal a lot of PMN with highly fragmented organisms. A transient T cell activation is seen in these cases both in the blood and in immunohistology.

Reversal Reactions and Lesions of Worsening/Relapse

The terms upgrading and downgrading reactions have been used by D.S. Ridley. The best instances of what this signifies are found in the description of the evolution of leprosy lesions (Ramanujam, 1978). The transformation to the lepromatous disease of the incipient lesions of childhood was in many instances by spurts of activity in the form of erythema and/or infiltration. There is progressive increase in the extent and number of lesions. The progress is insidious. This includes nerve involvement also. Bacteriological deterioration is observed. Waxing and waning of cellular immunity during spurts of activity may be found. Such a progression is seen among cases who are inadequately treated for a short time or where the treatment has been interrupted for a long time. Interestingly, relapses in treated cases of lepromatous or BL leprosy may be in the form of borderline leprosy, BT or BB subtypes. Fresh papules show AFB in smears.

Reactions of BT or BB types are acute in onset and occur during the first six months of treatment or six months after RFT. In cases which are subject to repeated reactions these reactions may occur even later. There is increase in erythema and swelling of lesions due to oedema. There is oedema of the surrounding area also. Sometimes this involves the hands and feet as well. Acute painful neuritis of previously involved nerves may occur. Fresh papular lesions, from pinhead to medium size, may be seen. Reacting lesions subside with scaling. The synovial bursae on the dorsum of wrist and ankles may be swollen. Lymphnode enlargement and joint effusions may be seen. Orchitis may be observed rarely. Paralysis is often sudden. Twenty per cent of cases have only predominantly skin lesions and trunk nerves escape. These are the usual ones where the relapse is manifested as a reaction and is often the first episode. If the initial condition was BT leprosy, skin smears are negative. If the condition of reaction is on account of sliding from BL to BB or BB to BT, the BI progressively diminishes. In upgrading BL reaction the lesions tend to get localised. There may be some amount of constitutional disturbances. ENL are not observed. Circinate lesions are characterised by an abrupt inner margin. Subsidence is with scaling. There is an appreciable fall in BI. In BT reactions nerve abscesses are observed after subsidence of acute neuritis.

What distinguishes the reactional from the active state is intense inter-cellular and sometimes intra-cellular oedema. There is heavy infiltration by plasma cells. This occurs in the backdrop of the particular type of borderline leprosy.

In the BT reactions the size of the Fernandez response to Dharmendra lepromin is greater than what one expects. The corresponding Mitsuda response is unaltered. In BB reactions, evidence of enhanced T cell responses was seen to M. leprae antigen whereas there was deterioration in the BT reactional patients (Nath and Laal, 1986).

Hyperactivity of the humoral limb of the immune system in the reactional states is denoted by increase in the levels of immunoglobulin and circulating immune complexes. Evidence of activation of the complement system is found in circulation and at sites of neuritis (Ramanathan, et al, 1985; Ramanathan, et al, 1969). They also lack the ability to metabolize immune complexes which is the distinguishing point between reactional and active states (Table 8.5).

TABLE 8.5: Summary of the Differences between Reversal Reaction and Relapse/Worsening

Reversal Reactions*	Relapse/Worsening
Observed in BT, BB, BL	Observed in subsided LL, LLs, BT, BB, BL
History	
Under treatment, within six months or later in recurrent reactions.	Treated in the long past, after six months during surveillance. Inadequately treated, i.e, MB given PB treatment.
As upgrading from BL-BB; BB-BT.	Downgrading from BT-BB and BB-BL.
Constitutional Symptoms	
Nil in BT, Mild in BL.	Nil, except when relapse occurs as reaction.
Signs	
Increase in erythema, swelling, tenderness on tapping or getting hurt. Succulent feel. Few fresh lesions with surrounding oedema, oedema of hands and feet.	Increase in extent. No oedema. Fresh lesions. No tenderness. Rubbery consistency. Oedema of hands and feet is rare.
BL get localised. In circinate lesions, inner border abrupt.	Lesions retain their morphology. Subside under treatment.
BB lesions become circumscribed with abrupt inner and outer borders. In severe reaction, ulcerations of lesions occur.	No ulcerations seen
Acute painful neuritis often present. Nerves exquisitely tender.	Fresh nerve involvement. No pain. Tenderness not marked.
Nerve abscesses may be found after subsidence.	No nerve abscess.
Lesions subside with scaling.	No scaling observed.
Systemic Involvement	
Lymphnode enlargement, joint and synovial effusion, rarely orchitis	Systemic involvement rare; seen if relapse manifests as reaction.
Smears of Skin for AFB	
Decrease in BI. Fresh lesions negative.	BI depends on subtype of leprosy. Fresh lesions positive if taken early.

(*Contd*)

Reversal Reactions*	Relapse/Worsening
Lepromin	Lepromin response corresponds to subtype.
In BT reaction Fernandez response pronounced. Mitsuda correspondingly less intense.	
T cell response enhanced in blood in BB and BL. Lowered in BT.	According to subtype.
CIC levels elevated, lack solubilization.	CIC solubilization not disturbed; antibody levels increased using SACT.
Histology marked by inter and intracellular oedema and plasma cells. BI decrease.	Cellular infiltrate corresponds to subtype. Plasma cell numbers not noteworthy.

* (Ridley, 1969).

REFERENCES

Arunthathi, S.; Jacob, M.; Chacko, C.J.G., 1988, A clinical study of primary neuritic leprosy. Abst. 13th Int. Lepr. Congr, Quad Coop. Sanitar. PO 313.

Chopra, N.K.; Agarwal, J.S.; Pandya, P.G., 1990, A study of relapse in a multidrug therapy project, *Lepr Rev.*, 61, p 157-162.

Grugni, A.; Nadkarni, N.N.; Kini, M.S.; Mehta, V.R., 1990, Relapses in paucibacillary leprosy after MDT: A clinical study, *Int J Lepr*, 58, p 19-24.

Iyer, C.G.S.; Balakrishnan, S.; Ramu, G., 1977, A comparison of low and conventional dosage of dapsone in lepromatous leprosy, *Lepr India*, 49, p 372-386.

Kanchana, M.V.; Lakshminarayana, C.S.; Narayanan, P.R.; Sengupta, U.; Sinha, S.; Ramu, G., n.d., [Increased antibody levels in BT leprosy] (to be published).

Katoch, K.; Ramu, G.; Ramanathan, U.; Sengupta, U.; Sreevatsa; Sharma, V.D.; Shivannavar, C.T.; Katoch, V.M., 1989, Results of a modified WHO regimen in highly bacilliferous BL/LL patients, *Int J Lepr*, 57, p 451-457.

Nath, I.; Laal, S., 1986, Dichotomy in immune responses of leprosy reactions, Proc. workshop on reactions, New Delhi, p 100.

Ramanathan, V.D.; Palande, D.D.; Ramu, G.; Prabhakar, R., 1989, An immunohistochemical study of neuritis in leprosy, Proc. 16th IAL Conf., Trichur. Abst. O. P. 25.

Ramanathan, V.D.; Sharma, P.; Ramu, G.; Sengupta, U., 1985, Reduced complement mediated solubilisation in leprosy patients, *Clin Exp Immunol*, 60, p 553-558.

Ramanujam, K.; Ramu, G., 1969, Wade's Histoid lepromatous leprosy : report of a clinical study, *Lepr India*, 41, p 176.

Ramu, G.; Desikan, K.V., 1988, A follow-up of Borderline Tuberculoid leprosy under sulphone monotherapy, *Indian J Lepr*, 60, p 26-33.

Ramu, G.; Ramanujam, K., 1974, Relapses in Borderline leprosy, *Lepr India*, 46, p 19-25.

Raval, S.N.; Sengupta, U.; Ramu, G.; Prabune, P.V.; Desikan, K.V., 1982, A study of continuous bacillaemia in borderline and lepromatous leprosy, *Lepr India*, 54, p 623-633.

Ridley, D.S. 1969, Reactions in Leprosy, *Lepr Rev*, 40, p 77.

Thomas, A.; Nagarajan, M.; Prabhakar, R.; Tripathi, S.P., 1990, Controlled clinical trial of two regimens in multibacillary leprosy, *Int J Lepr*, 58, p 272-280.

Touw, J.; Langerdijk, E.; Stoner, J.L.; Balehu, A., 1983, Humoral immunity in leprosy: Immunological antibody activity in various disease patterns. G and M antibody responses to M. leprae infection, *Infect Immun*, 36, p 885.

9

DRUG RESISTANCE IN LEPROSY

B.K. GIRDHAR

The drug dapsone has been in continuous use since its induction in leprosy some 35-40 years ago. The drug has been found to be extremely effective both clinically and in inhibiting multiplication of M. leprae in the mouse footpad. Till about a decade ago, dapsone was being freely used as monotherapy, in variety of doses, in all forms of leprosy and all over the world. In fact monotherapy with dapsone continued to be the practice despite the realization that the cavitary pulmonary tuberculosis could not be cured by any of the available anti-tubercular drugs given alone. The delay in application of combined chemotherapy in leprosy was on account of several factors. Of these, the important were the non-availability of tools to verify resistance and the extraordinary efficacy of dapsone. However, despite its powerful action against M. leprae, treatment failures were suspected and recorded by several workers.

Soon after, the mouse foot pad system was described (Shepard, 1960), occurrence of dapsone resistance was shown beyond doubt (Pettit and Rees, 1964). Initial estimates indicated that it was not a serious problem, as the prevalence (calculated from figures available from Malaysia) was around two per 1000 (Pearson, 1981). However, the situation seemed to have changed by 1977 as by this time it was suspected to have already become a significant problem (WHO, 1977). Since 1975, formal surveys of dapsone resistance have been undertaken in several parts of the world. These studies have confirmed that dapsone resistance is a worldwide phenomenon and is on the increase (WHO, 1982). Subsequent reports and surveys have also indicated that as a consequence, *de novo* infection with resistant M. leprae was present in the community (Girdhar, et al, 1978; Person, et al, 1977).

There are two types of drug resistance. The secondary or

acquired resistance which develops following inadequate chemotherapy and presents clinically as initial improvement followed by deterioration despite continued treatment. The other type of resistance is primary, which occurs in untreated patients and results probably from infection with drug resistant organisms that are spread/discharged into the environment by the patients who have relapsed with secondary resistance.

The basis of this resistance in M. leprae is not known since M. leprae in very large numbers cannot be obtained in vitro. Our understanding of resistance in leprosy is really an extrapolation of what we have learnt from resistance in M. tuberculosis. The process is considered to be basically a selection of naturally occurring resistant mutants which is a normal phenomenon in any large proportion of organisms. With administration of individual effective drugs, the susceptible population gets killed and eliminated, but the surviving resistant mutants continue to multiply, resulting in clinical signs of relapse. Patients, receiving regular treatment in full doses, relapse quite late and mainly with high degree of resistance. Whereas, those given low dose of drug or irregularly, relapse earlier and often with low or intermediate degree of resistance.

Unlike with some other chemotherapeutic agents, the resistance in M. leprae to dapsone is a multi-step phenomenon. Therefore, all grades or degrees of resistance are encountered. All the wild strains were found to be sensitive to levels lower than 0.0001 per cent DDS in diet before secondary resistance became a common phenomenon. Hence 0.0001 per cent DDS in diet is taken as cut off point. Organisms, that continue to multiply in mice, receiving this concentration of DDS are considered low degree resistant organisms, and those that are able to resist ten times this dose are taken as moderately resistant whereas those that multiply in mice given DDS in dietary concentration of 0.01 per cent are considered fully resistant.

Diagnosis of dapsone resistance, though very important, has in the present situation less practical utility than the treatment of resistant (relapsed) patients. This is because we now understand that it is much easier to treat all multibacillary patients as potential cases of resistance than to try to find who has or is incubating resistance. We now know that, if monotherapy is continued, a large proportion of patients will ultimately develop the problem. Therefore, bactericidal drugs are used in combination to prevent/treat drug resistance. This is based on the expectation, which is well proved experimentally in TB, that naturally occurring resistant M. leprae to one drug will be killed by the concurrent administration of other and *vice versa* with the result that probability of any viable bacterium remaining unkilled will be extremely low.

Likewise, if a patient who has organisms that are already resistant to one of the drugs, a third drug would do the same together with one to which the organisms are still sensitive. This is the basic principle for MDT. Thus if all the MB patients, whether fresh (untreated), partially or fully treated with full dose of DDS or irregularly treated with DDS in the past, are given MDT regularly the need for diagnosis of dapsone resistance in a programme becomes an academic exercise.

However, where diagnosis and confirmation of resistance is required in patients already on DDS treatment, the foremost thing is suspicion. Whenever a borderline/lepromatous patient, who has or had been taking dapsone self-administered (meaning thereby, where dose and regularity are suspect), presents with any fresh lesions together with signs of healing on other sites, doubt of DDS resistance must arise. More often, these fresh lesions are in the form of 'histoid nodules' but sometimes these could be plaques and occasionally diffuse localized or generalized infiltration.

Skin-smear examination affords the first proof of resistance. On comparison of skin smears from both apparently healed (shrivelled) areas and the suspected fresh lesions, a much higher B.I. and M.I. in the fresh lesions strengthens the diagnosis of relapse, suggestive of resistance.

For a definitive proof, mouse foot-pad testing is the answer. Since this facility is not available in most of the centres, a clinical trial may be undertaken. A supervised course of dapsone, either orally or parentrally (at least 300 to 400 mg weekly) is given. Periodically, clinical response is recorded every three to six months and repeat smears, as above, are made every one to three months. In drug resistant cases, several different patterns of response may be seen. Patients, who previously received full dose treatment, will show none or only partial response for a brief period and then deteriorate. Those previously on low dose or irregular DDS will show an initial good response that resembles drug sensitive patients. However, after some months, active lesions with elevated MI and an increase in BI may result.

The limitations of clinical trials are that the result may be delayed and the proof may require time from three months to five years. Further, such tests are suitable only for those patients who relapse with active new lesions with high MI. In field surveys, employing mouse foot-pad technique resistant strains have been isolated even from patients without clinical relapse.

The ultimate test, as of today, is the drug susceptibility testing in mouse foot-pad. Whereas this is an important and a reliable tool, it requires a certain minimum number of organisms, is cumbersome, and takes six to twelve months for the answer. The test being very demanding, is limited to a few centres only. Essentially the test involves inoculating $5X10^3$ to 10^4 organisms in hind foot-pad of four groups of at least six mice each. One group, i.e., control is fed on normal food without dapsone. The other three groups are given DDS in concentrations of 0.0001, 0.001 and 0.01 per cent in diet. Six to twelve months after inoculation, the mice are sacrificed and AFB harvested from the foot-pads. If no multiplication is observed in the control mice, it indicates that the proportion of viable organisms in the inoculum was too small. If, on the other hand, multiplication is observed only in the control mice and not in any of DDS fed animals, the conclusion is that the inoculum had viable but DDS sensitive bacilli. If multiplication of M. leprae is observed in some or all the drug treated mice, the strain is resistant and the degree of resistance is reflected by the highest concentration of the drug in diet that permits multiplication of M. leprae.

In exactly the same way by substituting other drugs, the susceptibility of strains to them can be determined. For interpretation of the results, however, some more aspects have to be considered. These include the definition of resistance to the drug and the critical proportion of resistant organisms as criteria of drug resistance.

For definition, the behaviour of wild strains is the most important. Though this has been well studied for DDS long before resistance became a serious problem, similar information is not available in case of other drugs. However, for practical purposes the following levels are taken to indicate resistance to respective drugs:

1. Dapsone (DDS) 0.0001%
2. Clofazimine (CLO) 0.001 to 0.0001 per cent (mixing is a problem)

3. Rifampicin (RMP) 0.03 per cent
4. Ethionamide or Prothionamide 0.01%

Data regarding magnitude/problem of resistance to other drugs is far from adequate to enable any conclusions to be made. This is on account of the fact that these drugs have not been used for enough time and as extensively as dapsone. During the seventies, these drugs were, however, used as monotherapy, for some time, in patients relapsing under DDS. Some of the relapsed patients were put on monotherapy with drugs, like RMP and CLO while others had these drugs together with a weak bactericidal drug, like thiambutosine. Since the regularity of intake of these drugs in all probability was not optimal, resistance was anticipated and indeed has been reported. Three groups of workers, one each from United States (Jacobson, et al, 1976; Hastings, et al, 1981), Paris (Gullpa-Lauras, 1984) and India (Sreevatsa, et al, 1984) have found occurrence of RMP resistance together with dapsone resistance. Likewise, CLO resistance among DDS refractory cases has been reported from Ethiopia (Warndorff-van Diepen, 1982) and South India (Kar, et al, 1986).

One way cross resistance between CLO and RMP in a laboratory strain of M. leprae has also been observed. Morrison reported that a laboratory RMP resistant strain was fully sensitive to CLO whereas CLO resistant strain responded to RMP (Morrison, 1972).

Belgian workers have reported and confirmed resistance to thioamides (Pattyn, et al, 1975). Cross resistance between thiacetazone and thioamides in tuberculosis is well known. It is therefore, feared that a similar possibility may exist in leprosy and this may render an effective tool useless even in hospital situations. (Pattyn and Colston, 1985)

In the recent years, several *in-vitro* tests have been proposed for assessing susceptibility of M. leprae to drugs. These tests have not been found to give reproducible results in other laboratories. Further, their correlation with mouse foot-pad has not always been good.

Whereas it is not difficult to diagnose secondary drug resistance in MB patients, it is very difficult to do so in PB patients. For one, distinction between relapse and reversal reaction is not clear and more important, there are no organisms to study the susceptibility. The only recourse is to follow the patient and if or when he becomes smear-positive (at least 3+) to do mouse foot-pad studies.

Diagnosis of primary resistance is more of an epidemiological investigation rather than of any interest to the patient. More often, it is a retrospective finding. From the clinical point of view, there are no indicators or pointers to suspicion of resistance. Those patients, who do not respond to an effective drug in a manner known for those with susceptible infection, need to be tested much the same way as secondary resistant patients.

Keeping various facts about resistance in mind, there has been a complete change in treatment of patients both from individual as also control point of view. In fact this change to MDT has not only helped to contain the problem of resistance, but has also emboldened the health managers to convert this programme to an eradication one with the hope that leprosy would no longer be a public health problem by the year 2000 A.D.

REFERENCES

Girdhar, B.K.; Sreevatsa; Desikan, K.V., 1978, Primary sulphone resistance: A preliminary report, *Lepr India*, 50, p 352-5.

Guelpa-Lauras, C.C.; Grosset, J.; Constant-Desportes, M.; Brucker, G., 1984, Nine cases of rifampicin-resistant leprosy, *Int J Lepr*, 52, p 101-2.

Hastings, R.C.; Jacobson, R.R., 1981, Rifampicin resistant leprosy, *Health Cooperation Papers*, 1, p 47-54.

Jacobson, R.R.; Hastings, R.C., 1976, Rifampicin resistant leprosy *Lancet*, p 1304-5.

Kar, H.K.; Bhatia, V.N.; Harikrishanan, S., 1986, Combined clofazimine and dapsone resistant leprosy A case report, *Int J Lepr*, 54, p 389-391.

Morrison, N.E., 1972, Antimycobacterial activity of phenazine compounds, *Int J Lepr*, 40, p 219-220.

Pattyn, S.R.; Colston, M.J., 1978, Cross-resistance amongst thiambutosine, thiacetazone, ethionamide and prothionamide with Mycobacterium leprae, *Lepr Rev*, 49, p 324-6.

Pattyn, S.R.; Rollier, M-T.; Rollier, R.; van Loo G., 1975, Sensibilite envers la dapsone, la sulfamethoxy-pyridazine, et l'ethionamide, de Mycobacterium leprae provenant de malades traites par ces substances, *Int J Lepr*, 43, p 356-63. (quoted from *Lepr Rev*, 56, 1985, p 265-278.

Pearson, J.M.H., 1981, The problem of dapsone-resistant leprosy, *Int J Lepr*, 49, p 417-20.

Pearson, J.M.H; Halle, G.S.; Rees, R.J.W., 1977, Primary dapsone-resistant leprosy, *Lepr Rev*, 48, p 129-32.

Pettit, J.H.S.; Rees, R.J.W., 1964, Sulphone resistance in leprosy: An experimental and clinical study, *Lancet*, i, p 673-4.

Shepard, C.C., 1960, Acid-fast bacilli in nasal excretions in leprosy and results of inoculation of mice, *Amer J Hyg*, 71, p. 147-57.

Sreevatsa; Girdhar, B.K.; Ramu, G.; Desikan, K.V., 1989, Parallel dapsone and rifampicin resistance: A Prospective Study, *Japanese J Lepr*, 53, p. 28-31.

WHO, 1977, *Expert Committe on Leprosy, Fifth report*, Tech. Rep. Series 607, World Health Organisation, Geneva.

WHO, 1982, *Chemotherapy of leprosy for control programmes*, WHO Study group, Tech. Rep. Series 675, World Health Organization, Geneva.

Warndorff-van Diepen, T., 1982, Clofazmine-resistant leprosy: A case report, *Int J Lepr*, 50, p 139-42.

10

MANAGEMENT AND MONITORING OF BACTERIOLOGICAL INDEX

V.N. BHATIA

Efficient services for the reporting of skin smears form an important component of MDT campaigns. Bacterial Index (BI) remains the most practical test for assessing bacteriological status of a patient in the field. It is essential that the uniformity and reliability of such an examination is maintained. In order to attain proficiency in reporting, the proper management and monitoring of BI is necessary.

What is BI ?

BI is a rough index expressing probable number of Acid-Fast Bacilli (AFB) for standardized microscopic field in the skin smear. If the smear is properly made, it may be indicative of the load of bacteria at the site from which the material was collected. BI may vary from site to site. Averaging BI mathematically may be misleading. BI does not differentiate living and dead bacilli. It is also not a reflection of total bacillary load in the body.

How to determine BI ?

It has been accepted to follow Ridley's scale in the NLEP activities for the sake of keeping uniformity at the world level. The scale consists of six grades (from 1+ to +6) :

0 = No bacilli in 100 fields
1+ = 1-10 bacilli in 100 fields
2+ = 1-10 bacilli in 10 fields
3+ = 1-10 bacilli in one field

4+ = 10-100 bacilli in one field
5+ = 100-1000 bacilli in one field
6+ = More than 1000 bacilli in one field

In conventional practice 100 fields are counted in low bacillary smears and 50 or even 25 fields for highly bacillated smears. Mostly a microscopist starts the examination from top and closes it as soon as he completes the requisite number of fields. This is fallacious as distribution of bacilli is never uniform and there may be cases where the top has no bacilli even though the smear is highly bacillated. We have encountered smears where whole smear was negative except one field which had a clump containing 124 bacilli. Similarly, leaving gaps when changing the fields during microscopic examination is erroneous. A quick scanning of the smear before starting detailed examination for reporting BI may be necessary to avoid anomalies.

Errors in reporting occur due to overlapping of grades under Ridley system. Thus the previous system of classifying PB and MB cases on basis of BI had to be abandoned. Follow up of patients on the basis of BI reports may give erroneous interpretations due to same reasons. Reporting BI one unit less or more in the marginal cases is possible even with honest and expert technicians. The physician should see previous slides himself in all the cases where doubts arise. The previous slides should be preserved as a permanent preparation for this purpose. Reporting number of bacilli on which BI report was based may be helpful.

Accuracy of Reports

Accuracy of the reported BI depends on quality of preparing, fixing, staining and reading of the smears. There are possibilities of false positive and false negative reports.

False Positive Reports

Reasons for false positive reports are as follows:

1. Precipitates in carbol fuchsin.
2. Saprophytic AFB from water or staining solutions.
3. AFB from previous slide if Koplin Jar is used for staining;
4. Carry over of AFB from previous smear if slides are reused

False Negative Reports

Reasons for false negative reports are as follows:

1. Wrong selection of sites.
2. Improper incision.
3. Smear is too thin.
4. Smear is too thick.
5. Inadequate fixation.
6. Too much blood in the material.
7. Prolonged or improper storage.
8. Overheating of the smear.
9. Inadequate staining with carbol fuchsin.
10. Very strong counterstain.
11. Erratic or inadequate screening.
12. Mistakes in labelling, coding/decoding, identification and false reporting.

Quality control, continuous supervision and monitoring are necessary to ensure that the high standards of reporting are maintained. Observer errors and reader variations can be avoided by standardized training, adequate supervision of laboratory technicians and cross-checking.

Cross-checking

All the positive slides and at least 10 per cent of negative slides chosen at random should be sent for cross-checking. The slides should be checked not only for BI report but also for quality of smear (shape, thickness, loss of material, staining quality, deposits, quality of counterstaining and wiping off of the material while removing the oil from the slides or due to rubbing of the slides during transport).

Monitoring of Services

The efficiency and proficiency of the bacteriological services should be monitored continuously. Simple and uniform system for monitoring the operational aspects of bacteriological services have to be developed. Inter- and intra-observer variations should be checked and the number of smears examined per day as against the number expected should be noted. The managerial lapses, attitude of the technician and possible mistakes in interpretation should be noted.

Supervision

Supervisory activities are an essential component of any health programme. The bacteriological services should be closely supervised by a competent technician or a specialist. There is no substitute for on-the-spot guidance. The technician should be told about the mistakes while preparing the smear and examining it. Theoretical coachings are not effective.

Operational Evaluation

Independent evaluation will be valuable if it is carried out by specialists or experts and observations are made by the experts themselves on the spot. Reports made on the basis of information collected through third persons do not help.

Standardized Methods

Briefly, the following points must be kept in mind by every technician to achieve standardization of the procedures:

1. Proper labelling, proper entries and correct identification of the patient.
2. Proper communication between the physician and the technician regarding sites (or part there of) to be smeared.
3. Explaining procedure to the patient and taking him into confidence.
4. Properly identifying the sites and cleaning the site thoroughly before taking smear.
5. Ensuring haemostasis. Giving proper incision and avoiding blood in the material.
6. Proper scrapping, carrying sufficient material to make a uniform round smear of nearly one cm diameter.
7. Spreading of the material with care. The smear should neither be too thick nor too thin.
8. Proper drying, fixation, storage in a box and proper transport.
9. Use of quality stains and cold method for staining.

10. Proper screening of slides. Examining 100 fields from top gives erroneous result; rough scanning of the whole smear is necessary.

Safety

It should be ensured that the skin smear procedure is safe to the patient and to the technician. As a precaution against AIDS (and Hepatitis) we may use disposable blades. The cost factor will have to be borne in mind. Other precautions, as for any infection, have to be followed. Working in an endemic area is no excuse for ignoring the safety precautions.

Managerial Aspect

Bacteriological services still remain a weak link in the programme. The reasons are related to managerial lapses. Staff is either not adequate or not sufficiently trained. There is no provision for on-the-spot guidance, supervision and monitoring of the work. Technician is usually blamed even though the mistake may lie with the doctor.

Timely and regular supply of requirements, like good quality binocular microscope, spare oil immersion lenses, proper immersion oil, slides in good numbers, pretested quality reagents, alcohol, spirit lamps and spirit, should be ensured; usually these items are in short supply.

BI in the Field

Standardized methods, as detailed above, should be followed for collection of material and spreading it over the slide. Round smears, neither too thick nor too thin, free from blood and of the size of one centimetre diameter are preferred. The spread in the pattern of onion peels is a common error with beginners. The art of smear preparation comes with practice and quality of smear depends on motivation and on-the-spot guidance of the technician.

A field kit for smear collection must be prepared. A stool, a work-bench and gas may not be available in the field. We have to compromise. It is possible to collect skin smears even under a tree. Necessary precautions, detailed above, should however be followed.

The substitute practices, possible problems and trouble shooting in the field should be discussed during training of the technicians.

Fixation

Fixation protects smear from damage during handling and preserves structure of the bacilli and cells. It also kills M. leprae. The smears must first be dried under a petri-dish and then fixed immediately over a jar containing formalin for fifteen minutes. Alternatively, slides with the smear facing up can be passed two to three times over a flame.

Storage

The fixed slides should be stored in a slide box in order to protect them from moisture, dust, insects and sunlight. If a wooden slide box is not available, cardboard container in which new slides are supplied can be used. A corrugated sheet of paper can be fixed on the sides to keep the slides in position. Covering the slide with black paper may protect the smears against adverse effect of sunlight.

Transport

Slides must be protected from breakage and rubbing against each other and against any other surface. Each slide should be wrapped in paper (preferably black). The whole bundle of slides should again be wrapped and packed tightly in a box. Both slides and the box should be protected by layers of some soft material, like cotton wool. The box should again be wrapped in a paper. The clinical details for each slide should accompany the slides.

MDT Campaigns in Low-endemic Areas

The programme does not have organised linkage with PHC system at present. The staff is not trained on the lines of NLEP strategies. The integration of NLEP with PHC needs quick preparation and rational approach at each level. Bacteriological back-up will, no doubt, be necessary. The training, re-training, orientation, post-training liaison and on-the-spot guidance may be necessary.

Although case load in low-endemic areas may be low, the

percentage of MB cases may be high. Moreover, every suspected leprosy case will have to be screened bacteriologically. The skin smears must be sent to the laboratories identified for the purpose.

The system of quality control, random checking of smear results and continuous supervision will have to be incorporated. The regional or reference laboratories for this purpose should be identified.

Training

It is essential to train control-programme personnel for taking smears of good quality in order to organize an efficient service for collecting and processing skin smears. Following steps in this direction need be taken:

1. Training, re-training and orientation courses may be necessary for technicians of Primary Health Care. Provision should be made for post-training liaison, continuous education and on-the-spot guidance. Special syllabi have to be developed for this purpose.
2. A working manual should be prepared for the guidance of all the staff involved in NLEP work. The modifications in the fields and in the non-endemic areas must be clearly specified.
3. All the modern teaching aids, like slide projector, over-head projector, etc., should be provided to the teachers. Funds must be allocated for this purpose. Many video films on leprosy have been made available to the training centres. Only a few may be suitable for training purpose.
4. Good teachers are either not available or not involved in NLEP. Even the best teachers may need re-orientation to changing needs of the programme. Involvement of medical colleges, other national institutes/centres and non-governmental organizations may be necessary.

BACKGROUND REFERENCES

Bhatia, V.N., 1987, Bacterial Index: Ridley's vs Dharmendra's scale, *Indian J Lepr*, 59, p. 80-83.

Bhatia, V.N., 1987, Skin smear examination in relation to multi-drug therapy campaigns, *Ind J Lep*, 59, p 75-79.

Bhatia, V.N., 1987, *Standardization of skin smear examination in leprosy: Proceedings of IAL Workshop held at GRECALTES*, Calcutta.

Bhatia, V.N., 1988, Importance of good quality skin smears to peripheral worker in leprosy eradication programme, *Ind J Lep*, 60, p 230-234.

Bhatia, V.N.; Sirumban P.; Padma M.N.; Harikrishnan S., 1986, Retrospective analysis of smear examination from multiple sites in multibacillary leprosy, *Ind J Lep*, 58, p 257-262.

Bhatia, V.N.; Vanaja, G.; Rao, S.; Enango, T.V., 1990, Some observations on skin smear examination, *Ind J Lepr*, 62, p 338-345.

Leiker, D.L.; McDougall, A.C., 1983, *Technical guide for smear examination for leprosy by direct microscopy*, Leprosy Documentation Service, Amsterdam.

NLEP, 1985, *Guidelines on case detection, treatment, follow up and reporting, National Leprosy Eradication Programme*, Government of India, New Delhi.

WHO, 1982, *Chemotherapy of Leprosy for Control Programmes: Report of a WHO Study Group*, Technical Report Series 675, World Health Organisation, Geneva.

11

FIELD MANAGEMENT OF DISABILITIES/DEFORMITIES

ERNEST P. FRITSCHI

It is indeed encouraging to note that the National Leprosy Eradication Programme (NLEP) is giving some attention to this very vital subject. This is not only for the sake of alleviating the intense human suffering caused by disfigurements and open sores due to the disease, but also for improving the image of leprosy in the mind of public which erroneously consider the deformed hands and feet as leprosy.

The field is the front line in the battle against increasing disability and deformity but it must be recognised that the "front" can only be sustained by an adequate back-up service which must be capable of supporting the assault. This paper therefore deals with the whole campaign, while stressing the front line situation.

Just as the starting point in the NLEP is the identification of patients in the community, so the first step in the care of the disabled is to identify the patients who are already manifesting some neurological deficit. There has been a great controversy as to whether anaesthesia should be regarded as deformity. I do not propose to touch on this controversy, but only to say that if we fail to warn the patient with anaesthetic hands or feet of the danger, then we miss the opportunity to prevent increasing disability and deformity.

Infrastructure

The key person in the detection, documentation and treatment of deformity is the Physiotherapy Technician who has undergone a nine months' course in leprosy physiotherapy. It is understood that often this post is not filled and when it is, there is no clear understanding by the whole team from the District Leprosy Officer (DLO) downwards what his specific role is.

If there is a physiotherapy technician available in the team, then our task is easy, if not available, it is necessary to train a Non-Medical Supervisor (NMS) in the techniques and assessments required. Orientation periods are also required for the Medical Officers (MOs) and DLOs as to the job-description of this person and his responsibilities and requirements to fulfil his tasks.

The first need that we face, therefore, is the role and definition of the physiotherapy technician.

The second is to make available a place of work, ideally in the twenty bed Temporary Hospitalisation Ward (THW), and the required equipment, instruments and supplies necessary for him/her to perform.

We shall now consider the problems which will be faced.

Problem 1: How do we identify at the earliest moment any new neurological impairment, sensory or motor?

Of great help in the identification of patients at risk, would be a serological test. One such test is currently been field tested in Nepal. This test identifies the patients in the BL area of the spectrum and is said to correlate well with the possibility of reversal reaction occurring in the patient. This test is not yet published (Theuvenet, *personal communication*).

At the present moment we have to rely on clinically detectable signs of impairment. The key person in this identification is the paramedical worker (PMW) who is the first and most regular team member to see the patient. He must refer the patient to the Supervisor, Physiotherapist and Doctor. It has been observed (Macaden, *unpublished communication*) in a carefully monitored Leprosy Control Programme that in the early stages of induction of patients into MDT regimens, a significant proportion of patients develop weakness particularly in the ulnar supplied muscles. This is not surprising as the impact of powerful anti-bacterial drugs is more than likely to increase local inflammatory reactions and thereby produce the internal entrapment syndrome.

The condition is frequently missed by most NLEP teams because the only person competent to recognise early muscle weakness is the

Physiotherapist who sees only cases referred to him.

Therefore, it is necessary to train the most peripheral workers to carry out a few basic tests every time they see the patient. Three very simple tests may be applied.

1. *Sensory*: Gently stroke the ulnar border of the palm of both hands: Does the patient feel the sensation on both sides equally? Repeat the test stroking the outer border of the thumb.
2. *Motor*: (4th palmar interosseus) Ask the patient to extend the fingers of both hands keeping the fingers together. Test for the ability to hold a piece of paper between little and ring fingers without bending the fingers.
3. *Abductor Digiti Minimi*: In the same position as above, is the patient able to move the little finger out against resistance without bending it equally on both sides?

If the field staff feels there is any weakness, the case must be immediately referred to the Physiotherapist for full assessment and referral to the MO. The patient is then admitted to the THW for treatment with a course of steroid. The MDT treatment need not be discontinued during the treatment of neuritis.

Problem 2: Assessment and management of established nerve paralysis.

This is the task of the Physiotherapist. Perhaps it will be most clear if expressed as a flow chart.

It is the duty of each DLO and/or MO to establish communication with any plastic, orthopaedic and ophthalmic surgeon whether Government or private in the area, who may be willing to examine/operate on leprosy patients. The DLO must also advise surgeons concerned as to where they can get guidance/training/experience in treating such cases.

The Physiotherapist must select and prepare cases for surgery and then look after them after operation. Without the possibility of specialist surgical services the Physiotherapist cannot be expected to function effectively.

Problem 3: The anaesthetic foot is always liable to produce corns, callosities, blisters and ulcerations.

Continual care has to be exercised by the patient to prevent these. The Physiotherapist is the most qualified member of the team for the purpose.

FLOW CHART : DEFORMITIES AND DISABILITIES

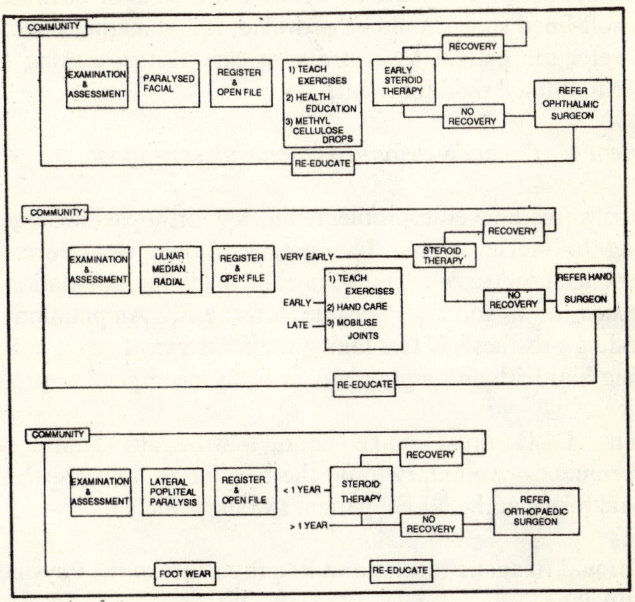

The following are the principles to be learned by the patient:

1. **Never stand when you can sit.**
2. **If only one foot is anaesthetic, never stand on that foot but only on the good foot.**
3. **Always use footwear. An undeformed anaesthetic foot can be kept unharmed simply by providing a well fitting soft insoled shoe or sandal with heel strap/counter and toe covers.**
4. **The anaesthetic foot must be examined systematically in proper light every day after bath. Discoloured areas, uneven thickening, blisters or small haematomata and open injury or penetrating**

thorn should be observed regularly.

A blister or haematoma requires complete rest for two days. Open wounds must be covered at least with an adhesive dressing. Penetrating thorns must be removed.

Uneven thickening of the skin must be trimmed, or soaked and scraped off.

5. The foot with a chronic ulcer must be treated with a plaster of Paris boot for at least six weeks and then after healing, a good soft-lined shoe should be provided. It is sometimes necessary to refer the patient to centre with expertise in making moulded MCR lined rigid footwears.

Problem 4: The badly deformed chronic ulcerated foot.

This is an orthopaedic problem, but few orthopaedic surgeons are willing to tackle them. The patient should be referred to an experienced centre or arrangements be made for amputation and the provision of a good serviceable prosthesis. Amputation without providing prosthesis is like taking the food away from a hungry man leaving him with an empty plate. It is an incomplete unprofessional service.

The DLO must make contact with any centre whether Government or voluntary to do the needful and the prosthesis must be paid for from the NLEP patient's welfare budget.

Additional Responsibilities and Requirements of the Physiotherapy Technicians

The physiotherapist must maintain a separate register of all the patients under his care, even when they are removed from the control. These ex-patient are recognised as leprosy patient by every man in the street. To treat them intelligently, conscientiously and humanely is a part of the responsibility of the NLEP.

For the Physiotherapist to be able to function properly, it is necessary to provide him/her with adcquate space and a supply of plaster of Paris, guaze, starch, etc., and a few instruments, gomometers, splints, etc. sufficient supply of oil for finger massage and if possible wax bath to be provided to him. All these items can be bought under the relevant budget head by the DLO as Secretary of the District Society. For this the funds are available, man-power is sanctioned, but what is required is motivation, boldness and a sense of duty on the part of those implementing the NLEP.

It is possible today not only to cure leprosy but also to prevent the inexorable increase in deformity and disability which is so demoralising to the ex-patient and his family. No eradication programme is complete without this service.

PART V

FACETS OF LEPROSY ERADICATION

12

ROLE OF SPECIALISED CENTRES IN LEPROSY CONTROL PROGRAMME

NAVNIT K. SHARMA

A specialised centre, e.g., the Department of Skin, V.D. and Leprosy in a Medical College, can contribute towards leprosy control in diagnosis, treatment and survey.

Diagnosis

As early diagnosis of disease constitutes the very basis of effective control, picking up of early cases is most important. In low endemic areas, the awareness of the disease is lesser and the stigma of the disease is very high. Therefore, either the person is not aware or he doesn't want others to know that he has got the disease. Early effects of the disease are produced and noticed on skin. So, the case is most likely to come first to Skin Out Patient Department (OPD) Therefore, it is very important to pick up such cases and institute proper treatment.

Secondly, many skin diseases have got lesions which are similar to those appearing during different stages of leprosy, e.g., hypopigmented macules, nodules, erythematours patches and nerve involvement. These may be confused with leprosy, wrongly diagnosed and treated by the field-worker. Such cases, naturally, do not respond to anti-leprosy treatment and constitute a problematic condition. These can be properly diagnosed and treated at the Specialised Centre.

Management

Unexpected course of the disease following treatment

Many problematic situations cannot be properly tackled in the field and the expected improvement does not occur. Such cases are referred to Specialised Centre for further management. These may include:

(i) Cases of initial wrong work-up and assessment,
(ii) Relapse,
(iii) Reactions, and
(iv) Dapsone-resistance.

Such cases need investigation and appropriate management after admission.

Complications due to disease

Some cases may have complications due to leprosy, e.g., ulcers, secondary infection of the cuts and wounds with bacteria and infestation with maggots. These cases cannot be managed in the field and have to be hospitalised.

Cases requiring surgical treatment

Some cases may have problems for which surgery is required, e.g., gangrene and correction of deformities. After surgical correction of deformities, physiotherapy is a must. This should be done under the supervision of surgeon in the Specialised Centre.

Associated problems and emergencies

As leprosy is a chronic disease with prolonged course, many patients may develop concurrent diseases due to other associated pathogenic factors, e.g., problems connected with ageing, like cataract, enlargement of prostate and loss of teeth, generalised problems, like diabetes, hypertension, coronary artery disease and chest-infections, and last but not the least, leprosy patients may be afflicted with medical, surgical, obstetrical and gynaecological emergencies, like any other group in the general population. For all these situations, not only does the patient need to stay in or close to a hospital, but the help of specialist(s) from other branches of medical sciences is also required.

Because of the stigma attached to the disease and the resultant disturbed psyche, the patient is not able to mobilise and get the support of the concerned specialist(s). The consultant, treating them for leprosy, needs to act as a resource person to mobilise the help of concerned specialists and arrange for admission of the patient in temporary hospitalisation ward (THW) for leprosy patients. It would be nice if machines and gadgets frequently used in this connection, e.g., ECG machine and X-Ray machine as also facilities for operations and physiotherapy are available in the leprosy unit of the department.

Education

All concerned with the handling of leprosy patients, in addition to the patient care need to be educated about the various aspects of the disease and their possible impact on contacts, family members and society at large. In this connection, the points, which need to be specially highlighted, are:

(a) Explanation of the present situation of the disease, that it is like any other infective disease and can be successfully treated;
(b) A patient of leprosy is not a leper for life;
(c) Except for a few cases, most of the leprosy patients constitute negligible or no risk of infection to others;
(d) Effective treatment is available to the patients. However, he should be punctual and regular in continuing it;
(e) Information about facilities available from the government agencies for treatment of leprosy patients, and the need for their being motivated to utilise them;
(f) The disease puts certain limitations on patients because of loss of sensations. So he/she should choose/modify work in the light of these;
(g) All efforts should be made to avoid injury and subsequent infections in order to prevent deformities and mutilations; and
(h) Last but not the least, the self-respect of the patient and the confidence that he/she will be alright and after treatment be a useful member of his society again has to be built up and sustained.

Besides these, the resident doctor, nursing staff and the attendant staff looking after leprosy patients also need to be given information on the disease, so that they do not carry any prejudice or unnecessary fear of acquiring the disease and hurt the feelings of leprosy patients, or lower their morale.

They should also be explained about the care of the patient, particularly about avoiding injury during transportation from one section of the hospital to another. The patient should not walk long distances bare-footed and should preferably be transported on a wheel-chair. Information may also be given on the disinfection of the used clothes, beddings and disposal of dressings.

Although it would be ideal for the doctor to give this education himself/herself, it would, however, be of help if a trained medical social worker is available for this. This would go a long way to make it a success and lessen the work load of the doctor in charge.

Besides these, efforts can also be made to educate general public and mobilise their support for organising/augmenting resources for treatment of leprosy patients and for approaching organised resourceful groups, like Indian Medical Association (IMA) Branches, Ladies' Clubs, Rotary Club and Lions Club. Survey work through organisation of skin camps in slum areas, factories and schools may also be done to detect and treat new cases of leprosy. Special efforts can be made to educate general public and inmates of the college campus on Leprosy Day observed annually on January, 30.

All these activities can be performed in the existing set-up by augmenting the already available resources for treatment of leprosy patients in the leprosy unit of the department.

13

MONITORING OF MDT IN ENDEMIC AND LOW-ENDEMIC AREAS

B.M.S. BEDI

Multi-drug Therapy (MDT) is the most significant development in the management of leprosy. Unfortunately even now we are continuing to use monotherapy which is admission of our failure in tackling this most important public health problem.

The tendency of National Leprosy Eradication Programme (NLEP) to take up only selective endemic areas under MDT coverage is perhaps an ideal example of double standard in our handling of health problems of the nation. There is no excuse to justify non-implementation of MDT in all areas and keeping it confined to the endemic districts.

The concept of endemic and non-endemic is not really applicable to leprosy because no surveys have been conducted of late and all data is based on State reports which are not really representative of the actual state of affairs.

The world shall certainly not forgive this lapse because in present times monotherapy has no place even in low-endemic areas.

In endemic areas we do have some infrastructure of NLEP in the form of (a) SET Centre, (b) Leprosy Cell, (c) PMW/NMS, (d) DLO, and (e) SLO, and the government has laid down stringent and meticulous plans for detection of new cases and monitoring of treatment of the known cases. There PMW/NMS is the key person who keeps records of the follow-up, clinical and bacteriological improvement which is being reported to DLO and SLO. Monthly figures are compiled and sent to Directorate General of Health Services and data is thus compiled at level of Ministry of Health and the same is circulated to WHO, VOs, etc.

This system is fully documented with detailed records but has many lacunae and pitfalls for example –

(a) The whole foundation of the progress is founded on efficient PMWs/NMSs who may not always come up to the standard expected of them especially when many of them have no detailed background of protean manifestations of disease, differential diagnosis and side effects of drugs being used.
(b) MOs and DLOs have not been always updated on present status of disease and its manifestations. Moreover, they are not willing participants always but made to occupy this role by force of circumstances. Therefore, they lack the desired motivation and are content to just mark their time and to countersign and forward the documents passed over by the PMW/NMS.
(c) The present concept of targets in detection, discharges, money incentive, etc., may seem good on paper but the emphasis seems to be more on statistics with the result that tinea versicolour cases are being included in new detection series and random discharges are indicated on the paper to meet the given targets. The incentive scheme seems to be backfiring and thus giving distorted dimensions.
(d) The part-time roving consultants who are appointed on regional basis lack the requisite authority and they, being usually retired, are wanting in necessary drive, desire, determination and dynamism. They play the role of Public Relation Officer (PRO) of the programme.
(e) The national evaluation of the programme has already revealed many of the above pitfalls because results show over-enthusiasm in meeting targets rather than control or eradication of disease.

Low-endemic Areas

Here, the requisite infrastructure is woefully lacking and the detection and treatment is given secondary place. Monotherapy still continues and drug resistant cases keep emerging.

The programme is linked with PHCs and multipurpose workers and MO and CMOs lack necessary orientation on the clinical aspects of the disease.

They are given periodic refresher courses but they, being preoccupied with other multifarious health activities, leprosy takes a back seat in their priorities.

Due to lack of experience, many full blown lepromatous leprosy cases are diagnosed as urticaria and are treated with corticosteroids which further mask the signs and symptoms until the disease progresses to an advanced stage when deformities become inevitable.

The infrequent positive smears also do not give the technician enough experience in laboratory smear preparation.

The lack of home visits precludes proper follow up of even existing cases.

Perhaps the useful activity is centred only on Urban Leprosy Centre (ULC) or State Leprosy Centres (SLC) or Medical Colleges.

The result of migration of population has caused influx of lepromatous leprosy cases into low-endemic areas thereby posing further challenge to the existing approach of separating the country into endemic and low-endemic areas.

Periodic shortage of essential drugs sometimes enforces disruption of treatment.

The remedy lies in strengthening the infrastructure, increasing the training, job satisfaction and motivation of workers, and perhaps in a national approach to this problem, otherwise low-endemic areas of today shall soon become endemic. There should be proper linkage of leprosy eradication programme with all medical colleges.

14

ROLE OF URBAN LEPROSY PROJECT IN A COSMOPOLITAN CITY IN THE CONTROL OF LEPROSY

R. GANAPATI

An urban area is a highly artificial situation where human beings have learnt to mutually exist. The rapidity of urbanization in countries endemic for leprosy has posed special challenges to those attempting to control leprosy by the delivery of Multi-drug Therapy (MDT).

Under National Leprosy Eradication Programme (NLEP), MDT is being implemented in a phased manner since 1981. The achievements in some of the districts are very encouraging, thus indicating possible eradication of leprosy.

Due to rapid industrialization and population migration to urban areas, especially metropolitan cities, such as Bombay, Calcutta, Delhi and Madras, the size of the problem is also gradually shifting to these areas. Hence, it is questionable whether effective eradication could be achieved in districts if these metropolitan cities are not brought under a special programme.

Planning for MDT Programme

In view of population heterogenecity due to multiplicity of socio-economic strata, variable prevalence rates among slums and non-slum population, complex health services and incoordinated functioning of voluntary organizations engaged in leprosy service, an ideal solution rests in an integrated approach to deliver MDT by involving all the health agencies – government, municipal and private. A good co-ordination between leprosy agencies and non-leprosy agencies is essential. There is a need to gather data on all health services available including non-leprosy agencies in addition to leprosy control programmes in operation in any urban area before launching MDT programme.

For the purpose of better planning and implementation of MDT in cities, it is advisable to classify cities according to the following criteria based on population:

1. *Megalopolis (Super-urban) with Population more than eight million:*

   (i) Greater Bombay, (ii) Greater Calcutta including Howrah, and (iii) Greater Delhi.

2. *Metropolitan Areas with Population four to eight million:*

   (i) Bangalore, (ii) Hyderabad, and (iii) Madras.

3. *Cities with Population one to four million:*

   (a) Hyperendemic: (i) Kanpur, (ii) Nagpur.
   (b) Low-endemic: (i) Ahmedabad, (ii) Jaipur, (iii) Lucknow, and (iv) Pune.

4. *Cities with Population less than one million*, but where the problem of leprosy is keenly felt judging from published reports*:

   (i) Allahabad, (ii) Bharuch, (iii) Chandigarh, (iv) Cochin, (v) Coimbatore, (vi) Gwalior, (vii) Jodhpur, (viii) Kolhapur (ix) Ludhiana, (x) Madurai, (xi) Nasik, (xii) Solapur, (xiii) Surat, and (xiv) Vishakapatnam,

5. *Recently developed industrial complexes:*

   (i) Ankleshwar, (ii) Bhilai, (iii) Bombay — Pune, (iv) Bokaro, (v) Dhanbad, (vi) Kanpur, and (vii) Vapi

* Some of these cities might have crossed the million mark by now.

The problems faced by major cities in other parts of the world, like Manila, Rangoon, Rio, Sao Paulo and Mexico city have not been looked into. It was at the International Leprosy Congress in Bergen that the recommendation on the need for research in urban leprosy was first made. However, till today not many academic studies in urban areas from different parts of the world have been documented. For the first time, Indian Association of Leprologists held a seminar on urban leprosy control, in Bombay in 1974. In fact, urban leprosy is the youngest speciality in the field and it is still in its infancy.

Author's experience of MDT administration in Bombay with population levels now exceeding ten million, indicates that urban logistics have to be taken into consideration carefully:

1. Slum-dwellers who form nearly 50 per cent of Bombay's population and are a large reservoir of Mycobacterium leprae (mean prevalence rate of leprosy is approximately ten per 1000 with MB prevalence rate being one per 1000).
2. Artificial situations, like leprosy colonies with abnormally high concentration of the sources of infection.
3. Patients residing in other situations, like tenements and on pavements.

This calls for planning field identification and treatment delivery procedures which would ensure follow-up for periods as long as eight years for MB cases – three years treatment phase on an average to obtain bacterial negativity plus five years follow-up phase as per current recommendations. However, experiments on Fixed Duration Treatment (FDT) indicate possible drastic reduction in treatment periods. Nevertheless, surveillance period would still have to be very long, as relapse rates after FDT are still not clear.

Is the population unstable or "floating"? Questionnaire studies in Bombay show that nearly 75 per cent of the slum population and 97 per cent of leprosy patients continue to stay in the slums for more than six years. Three hundred families are said to migrate daily to Bombay, and these are reported not to leave Bombay. Thus, it is evident that the population is not very mobile.

With limited resources it is best to identify and treat the index infectious cases rather than attempt to unearth all early PB cases in the community. We have tried various experiments in leprosy colonies in order to reduce the bacillary load. In one colony we treated the MB cases only with WHO recommended MDT, and examined annually the healthy persons living in the colony. This experiment brought down the new case detection rate to very low levels. All the MB patients, who were treated from 1982, have been rendered negative. We have found that patients with a BI of more than 3+ do very poorly even after five years of MDT while such patients under FDT (24 months) have performed as well or even better. Under urban conditions it appears best to treat patients with a BI of 3+ and more as a separate group.

Integration of Leprosy with General Health Services (GHS)

Our operational research shows that in urban areas, leprosy services should not be isolated but should be linked up with the GHC system available. Leprosy today is ready to be accepted by the non-leprosy sector. If we do not integrate soon, the situation in the cities located in hyperendemic areas may go beyond our control.

Many rural leprosy hospitals in hyperendemic parts of the world have good facilities and the expertise to offer ideal deformity care including surgery and institutional rehabilitation. Deformity prevention methods are also practised in the field in some of the rural programmes. With the leprosy problem currently increasing in urban areas, there is a great need to provide for disability prevention and management. With some resourceful approach on the part of leprosy programme managers, it may be possible to harness the potentials available in general hospital facilities. Some city hospitals, especially those attached to medical colleges, have well developed speciality of plastic surgery. Cannot one use the surgeons in these centres for reconstructive surgery? If an urban leprosy programme (ULP) could have effective linkages with such centres instead of planning its own surgical facilities, considerable cost reduction and the object of integration will also be achieved. It has been found that trained Physiotherapy Technicians for pre-operative and post-operative physiotherapy may have to be provided to assist the surgeons in such instances.

It is needless to point out the evils of institutionalised rehabilitation for leprosy patients in the modern era when the concept of community-based rehabilitation (CBR) for all the physically handicapped is being introduced. An urban set-up is ideally suitable for the application of the CBR concept in which a leprosy patient is also included. A domiciliary approach, through offering of loans to leprosy patients for self-employment or placement of the leprosy handicapped in open industry with the liberalization of certification for fitness, has been reported to be successful.

With the proliferation of vocational rehabilitation centres for training as well as employment of the physically handicapped in big cities, there is scope for inclusion of leprosy in such centres. Any attempt to integrate leprosy in this manner should be preceded by health education (HE) of administration staff as well as other personnel in the centres concerned.

Success achieved in some areas in the integrated rehabilitation of leprosy patients may not imply that such techniques could be universally applied. However, there is a need for a thorough discussion on the possibility of persuing such measures under varied urban conditions.

Co-ordination

It is found that in many large cities multiple voluntary agencies – international as well as national – are operating field programmes and adopting well defined areas for their leprosy control work. In the same local government or city corporation units also may be functioning. Hence, it is essential that various units should co-ordinate their activities periodically in order to avoid duplication of work. Occasionally, an attitude of ego on the part of some programme managers is noticeable which may have to be subdued in the larger interest of patient services. Co-ordination meetings may help to resolve any conflicting issues among units.

15

HEALTH EDUCATION FOR EARLY DETECTION OF LEPROSY

A.B. HIRAMANI

Leprosy is a disease which is looked down upon not because it kills the patient or is highly contagious but because it disfigures the body, thereby attracting social stigma, borne out of unfounded and irrational beliefs about the disease. It is really unfortunate that, ever since the discovery of the disease, society has not been able to remove the concept of social stigma attached to leprosy. By removing this concept, we could have possibly been successful in removing the feeling of fear which acts as an impediment in the success of the programme. Many facets and phases of the National Leprosy Eradication Programme (NLEP) in India have so far not been able to remove this concept. The concept has overriding relationship with cognitive behaviour of the individual as far as leprosy is concerned. The disease can be treated and cured by medical intervention but psycho-social elements attached with the disease can be dealt with only by education to the individual, the family and the community.

There can be more intensive health education strategy for leprosy programme, considering an onslaught of the disease, its continuum, control and eradication. The World Health Organisation emphasized two important points to be included at all states of health education in leprosy (WHO, 1960):

(1) That it is to the advantage of the individual to have any suspicious lesion examined by somebody competent to do so; and
(2) that it is to the advantage of the patient to follow the advice given about attending regularly for treatment and doing those things which will prevent the development of disability or deformity.

As far as HE for early detection is concerned, our emphasis should be more on the first point made by the WHO. HE approach for early detection has to be 'one shot' and quick because the situation is such that the individual has, in real sense, not been affected by the disease. And in case, there are symptomatic features, then guiding for and providing early treatment to the affected individual will prevent the development of the disease.

It is, therefore, the individual and the community that have to be made aware of and prepared to realise the need of early detection of the disease. The traditional approach so far adopted in health education is that only health worker working in the leprosy programme or the health worker in general is responsible for educating the community. The approach of health education followed now is both, formal and informal education of the individual, family and the community. Under the informal approach, either the health worker or those personnel who are responsible for health education in the programme deal with the individual and the community in a very informal situation, and disseminate the health information. Nevertheless, this approach, although informal in nature, is generally turned into formal approach by health worker. Under the formal approach, the information on the disease aspects is disseminated through various channels such as print material, electronic media, and personal talks or counselling. The effectiveness of these media, however, depends upon multiple factors, such as, the need of the community, type of information given, and suitability of media of communication itself.

The health education strategy to achieve maximum output in early detection of cases of leprosy are discussed under three broad aspects:

(i) What are the channels of health education?
(ii) Who should organise health education?
(iii) Who are the target groups?

Channels of HE

(a) *Radio broadcasting*:

It is perhaps the least expensive method of mass communication as no new investment is required. With easy availability of transistor set, which is an inexpensive item, it has covered almost entire population. Software can be prepared by the experts on this subject keeping in view the needs, the cultural background and the literacy status of the community. Those programmes, which have repeated value, can be taped and replayed as and when required.

(b) *Films*:

Films not only provide entertainment but also provide education to the larger population. Educational films, followed by a small spell of entertainment programme, have been found more effective in creating interest among the public. However, it should be kept in mind that this should sustain the interest of the audience and maintain the tempo of the public towards understanding the message conveyed therein.

(c) *Press*:

The use of newspapers and magazines in India is still restricted to relatively small size of population as this is mostly used by the literate group. Some of the facets of the programme need to be made 'newsworthy' to seek press coverage and press support. Although the press may not have direct bearing on the programme as such, it will certainly help disseminate the information.

(d) *Printed Material*:

Like newspapers, print material including exhibits has also limited scope, but its impact cannot be discarded simply on the ground that the target group is not literate. In the community, printed material in the form of posters, leaflets, folders, slogans and exhibitions carrying simple but scientific and adequate knowledge can be used for both illiterate as well as literate population who in their own way will become transmitters of the message.

(e) *Folk Media*:

Fold media such as traditional plays, songs, music and puppet shows can be utilised; as the people find in this media a kind of information which is generally absent in the modern sophisticated media. Traditional folk media are generally suited to the people with low literacy and to those who are not yet exposed to cross cultural currents and new communication media. Without disturbing the traditional and cultural ways of behaviour of the tribal people, a suitable communication programme through tribal songs and plays can be prepared locally.

(f) *Television (TV)*:

As a means of communication, TV is a revolutionary step despite its complexity. Its potential in helping to bring about social change is immense. The programmes telecast on the *Doordarshan* in India have been found to be much effective. Nevertheless, it has some limitations when we use it in the population characterised by cultural and language diversity.

(g) *Inter-Personal Channel of Communication*:

Human nature, which is influenced by its social and cultural norms, is modified or changed to a great extent by inter-personal interaction. External and impersonal source of communication, although effective, do not effect the individual to the same extent as with personal or face to face communication. The listener has a direct control over the communicator who is responsible to satisfy the clients' query and thus obtain maximum motivation to understand and act in a desirable way.

While adopting the strategy of health education in early case detection, the involvement of the patient, family members and all those who matter for the community needs to be obtained at various stages.

Health Education by Whom?

Although it is primarily the job of health educator, we cannot depend for imparting the education about the disease only upon the health educator, who along with other responsibilities, may not be able to carry out the expected role as health educator in the field of leprosy. It is, therefore, necessary that the following personnel may also be utilised for health education:

(i) Health worker, including doctor,
(ii) Family members,
(iii) Community leaders,
(iv) School teachers and students,
(v) Members of the Mahila Mandals, and
(vi) Members of the Youth Clubs.

Health Worker is a formal member of the health team who, in most of the cases, resort to impersonal communication, however Health Workers enjoy the confidence of the community because of their being in regular touch with the latter. Health education approach used by them proves to be effective in a given situation. WHO also subscribes to this view. It recommends that "The chief impact on the public will, of necessity, be made by the paramedical personnel and social workers for it is they who will go into the homes of the patients and the general public." (WHO, 1960). On the other hand, health education through family, community leaders, Mahila Mandals (ladies clubs), youth clubs, etc., is offered in a face to face situation and in an informal way. The situation in such health education process is that the communicator or educator, being the member of the same primary group, has much scope to monitor a change in the behaviour of the individual, and to pursue him to do what is desirable and advantageous to him. However, it needs to be seen that the educator has scientific knowledge of the subject to offer to the members. The school teacher and students have an unique relationship which can be said to be both, formal as well as informal. Teaching health aspects to the students in a learning situation, the teacher is able to pass on the knowledge and to point out possible consequences of the disease. It can help create positive or negative models and examples that will facilitate bring about behavioural changes. But health education teaching in the school has its limits. We must recognise that it is difficult to influence human behaviour, especially at an adult age. Therefore, health education through a teacher to a student at an early stages of education will have more influence.

While preparing health education material which is directed to be disseminated through various channels, the content ought to be very simple, scientific and acceptable to the community. In health education process, one has to use a variety of media because every media has its limitations, advantage and disadvantage in a particular situation. Although the formal channels of health education are considered to be useful, and effective, the most effective is the personal communication. Nevertheless, selection of media of health education needs to be judged from the point of view of the needs of the people and their choice.

REFERENCES

FCHE, 1991, *Health Education Policy Development and Processes and Structures*, Sixth International Seminar on Health Education, Bergneustadt, 22-26 June 1991, Federal Centre of Health Education.

Rosen, G., 1961, Evolving Trends in Health Education, *Canad J Public Health*, 52, December, p 499.

WHO, 1969, *Second Report of Expert Committee on Leprosy*, Technical Report Series, 189.

16

STRATEGY FOR LEPROSY ERADICATION PROGRAMME IN LOW-ENDEMIC AREAS

R.S. MISRA

India is a developing country having vast territory and a large population with a total of one-third of world leprosy patients, i.e., approximately three millions (Appendix 15). The country is divided into 25 States and six Union Territories. The economic, social and geographic factors vary from place to place and these affect the epidemiology of leprosy and the efficacy for implementing eradication measures.

India is one of the countries where the Eradication Programme is completely aided by the government by providing full support to strategies aimed at controlling leprosy. The present goal is to achieve total eradication of the disease by the year 2000 A.D. With a view to achieve this goal, the government is channelising all efforts through the National Leprosy Eradication Programme (NLEP) first launched in 1954, and through other voluntary agencies rendering yeoman's service to the cause of leprosy. Under the NLEP, the country is currently divided into high or hyper-endemic States having more than ten cases of leprosy per 1000 population, moderately endemic areas with five to ten per 1000 population and low-endemic States with prevalence less than five per 1000 population. NLEP is a vertical programme which provides all facilities relating to detection, treatment, surveillance and health-education (HE) in the high-endemic States. With the introduction of multi-drug therapy (MDT) and the resources available under the aegis of NLEP, many of these high endemic States have registered a notable decline in the disease (Table 16.1).

TABLE 16.1: District Registering Marked Decline in Endemicity

Ganjam (Orissa)	Vadodara (Gujarat)
North Arcot (Tamil Nadu)	Vijayanagram (Andhra Pradesh)
Purulia (West Bengal)	Wardha (Maharashtra)

Besides the high endemic areas, there are the low-endemic States and Union Territories (Table 16.2), and other States with pockets of low endemicity (Table 16.3). The rapid increase in population and its attendant problems of employment, housing, urbanisation and movement of tourists are factors insidiously operating in the spread of disease in these States. Migration of population across international borders from neighbouring countries, like Nepal and Bangladesh also account for the additional cases seen in the region – a situation similar to that occurring in Pakistan in transient phase (Pfau, et al, 1986). Furthermore, these areas do not fall under the vertical programme of NLEP and thus are grossly at disadvantage *vis-à-vis* endemic areas. Present reports indicate that the disease prevalence in some of these States is on the rise. In metropolises, like Delhi, the ever- increasing number of slums and resettlement colonies may prove to be major health hazards as seen in other cosmopolitan cities. (Revankar, et al, 1986). Unless we devise a system to tackle the problem in these areas, even the control of leprosy will remain incomplete – a far cry from its eradication. An attempt has been made to identify the problem in the low-endemic States and to suggest feasible measures for implementation.

TABLE 16.2: Primarily Low Endemic States/UTs (Below 5/1000)

States	UTs
Assam	Chandigarh
Goa, Daman and Diu	Dadra and Nagar Haveli
Haryana	Delhi
Himachal Pradesh	
Jammu & Kashmir	
Meghalaya	
Mizoram	
Rajasthan	
Tripura	

TABLE 16.3: States with Pockets of Low Endemicity

Arunachal Pradesh	Maharashtra
Gujarat	Manipur
Karnataka	Nagaland
Madhya Pradesh	Uttar Pradesh

Present set up and existing problem

Basic health services in low-endemic areas are provided through primary health centres and subcentres in rural areas, and in urban places this is done by municipal, voluntary and government dispensaries, general and medical college hospitals. In only some of these centres, there exists a paramedical worker (PMW) for leprosy, otherwise, the entire work is done by the staff engaged in delivering general health care.

The main problems faced are:

(a) Most of the reports on prevalence of leprosy from low endemic areas are based either on voluntary reporting by the patients themselves or on very old surveys that need to be updated. Hence the true prevalence of leprosy in these areas, which only can be an important guideline in formulating the measures for disease control, yet remains to be known, . This was evident from our study of the prevalence of leprosy in Delhi (Misra, et al, 1987).

(b) Amongst the people in low-endemic areas, a higher social stigma prevails against the disease as compared to endemic areas, and this in turn leads the people to hide their disease till it results in deformities.

(c) In the absence of proper follow up, even the few patients, who are put on therapy do not take the treatment regularly and completely. Added to this is the problem that MDT has not been uniformly introduced all over the country and many take monotherapy in the absence of proper supervision which is neither good for themselves nor for the success of NLEP, because of multiplication of primary and secondary drug resistance.

(d) Both the medical and paramedical staff have not received the necessary training to deal with the problem of leprosy.

Consequently, they are neither able to educate the patients about their problem nor give them the much needed encouragement to make them take the drugs properly and regularly. Early leprosy cases can easily be missed by the untrained person who does not have sufficient knowledge about the diesease. This is purely a practical problem and can only be corrected by adequate training at specialised centres.

(e) The health personnel in these areas do not find enough time to devote exclusively to the problem of leprosy. Further, absence of initiatives and incentives add to this dismal picture. Having no facility available at their disposal and due to financial constraints they are not in position to help the patient to seek proper advice elsewhere.

(f) For a disease rooted with strong stigma and prejudice health education of the community is an imperative adjunct to therapy. The best way to control the spread of leprosy is to encourage voluntary reporting and this can only be brought about by educating the community about the various social aspects of the disease to dispel the prevalent myths.

SUGGESTED MEASURES FOR CONTROL OF LEPROSY IN LOW-ENDEMIC AREAS

I. Provision of Training Facilities

This forms an integral part of our attempts to promote measures for control of leprosy. This infrastructure must be well built because this will reflect upon the type of service delivered in future. The problem should be solved at two major levels:

1. *Medical Curriculum*:

This involves the incorporation of various aspects of leprosy in the teaching curriculum, and the teaching and training in this field must be as practical as possible. The undergraduates must be shown the various clinical forms of the disease and simple techniques of testing for sensations, nerve and muscle function, of making smears and of learning to recognise the morphology of the bacilli. This must be accompanied by practical demonstrations and to drive home these facts the students must have compulsory training of ten to fifteen days in leprosy in the dermatology department of their medical colleges. During this period, they must be individually shown and asked to examine the cases of leprosy by experienced senior people in the speciality to improve their index of suspicion for leprosy. Assessment of adequate knowledge of leprosy should be an integral part of undergraduate medicine examination.

Postgraduates in the speciality should be told of the need for maintaining regular follow up in a proper manner. They should be made to prepare the slit smears and to read the bacteriological index themselves. A specific part of the qualifying test paper must include questions on leprosy. Wherever possible, students may be allotted projects in leprosy for their thesis or dissertation, so that they are exposed to the potential areas of research.

2. *Paramedical Staff*:

This forms an important part of the programme and include the following:

(a) Laboratory technician should receive adequate training to interpret the BI and to grade them so that the therapy can be appropriately monitored. The proper method of taking of slit smears must be taught by on-the-spot guidance, supervision and monitoring of the work (Bhatia, 1991).

(b) Nursing staff must also be given comprehensive training in diagnosis and management and in rendering proper advice to the patients and their families. Dressing trophic ulcers, and care of insensitive hands and feet during the course of follow-up should fall under their supervision and care.

(c) Rehabilitation workers must treat leprosy patients at par with other physically handicapped individuals and be in a position to give suitable advice to patients with resultant paralytic deformities and manage them independently. This includes provision of proper footwear, splints and other appliances, where necessary, to those with impending nerve paralysis. Trained workers from previously high-endemic areas, which have since become non-endemic, can be employed in these low-endemic areas.

II. Inservice Training of Health Personnel

The in-service training of both medical and paramedical personnel, will enable them to keep themselves abreast, update their knowledge with recent trends and to review their working techniques so that the method of work in these areas is under constant surveillance and the interest of the personnel is maintained. Emphasis must always be on such theoretical knowledge which is directly applicable to routine practice. Special problems faced in field by the staff can be discussed in workshops and seminars, and be sorted out in a manner that can be effectively carried out under the prevailing conditions.

III. Primary Health Centres (PHCs)

PHCs responsible for delivering health care in the rural areas must have a Medical Officer (MO) who, in addition to performing routine duties, has also been trained in leprosy work which includes diagnosis, monitoring of MDT, management of complications, and referrals to specialised centres when needed. These MOs must fix particular day and time of their work schedule to exclusively see patients of leprosy. They would also be responsible for maintaining statistics and supplying it to district administrators, and also ensuring a regular follow up and surveillance.

IV. Dermatology Departments of Medical Colleges/District Hospitals

Para-medical workers (PMWs) must be provided to the dermatology departments in urban areas. Doctors working in these departments must be urged to submit a monthly report on the number of patients under their treatment and of those declared cured. It has also been shown in urban areas that with effective guidance and encouragement to doctors working in government dispensaries or even to those engaged in private practice, a significant number of leprosy patients can be benefited (Revankar, et al, 1982). These doctors should also receive incentives for leprosy work at par with staff working in the vertical programme.

V. Referral Centres (RCs)

RCs with facilities for delivering expert care under one roof, must be established. These centres should have temporary hospitalisation wards (THW) to admit serious cases of reactions and complications, rehabilitation centres and reconstructive surgery units. Such centres attached to big hospitals and medical colleges should be restricted in number to suit the financial constraints. Patients from distant places in the region may be provided financial assistance to attend these centres when needed.

VI. Health Education of the Community

In short, our entire strategy in low endemic areas starts as shown in the Fig. 16.1 by encouraging maximum cooperation from the community, PMWs and the health personnel in rural and urban areas. The specialised centre is the nucleus which caters to the patients referred to them from the periphery.

In certain situations, especially in mountainous regions, where leprosy is prevalent it may be difficult for both the patient and the PMW to take or to give benefit of treatment respectively. An economically feasible method found successful by health authorities in China was either to reward the person for voluntary reporting or the PMW for bringing the patient under therapy (Haide, et al, 1982). These suggestions, with minimal financial constraints, may also be of use in other countries where only the endemic population has been well covered so far.

The problem of leprosy in low endemic areas can no longer be ignored because in terms of numbers it covers a population of 400 million, i.e., half the people of the country who are at risk. It will not be prudent to put it off for the future till such time that these areas also become hyperendemic due to proliferation of primary and secondary drug resistance to DDS. Financial constraints do not permit us to implement the vertical programme which may also not be completely desirable. Low prevalence of the disease itself keeps up the high social stigma and is responsible for ostracisation of the leprosy patient. With persistent health education a change in social attitude and practice of the people is to be brought about, fully supported by a committed political will to improve the economic and living conditions of the economically backward.

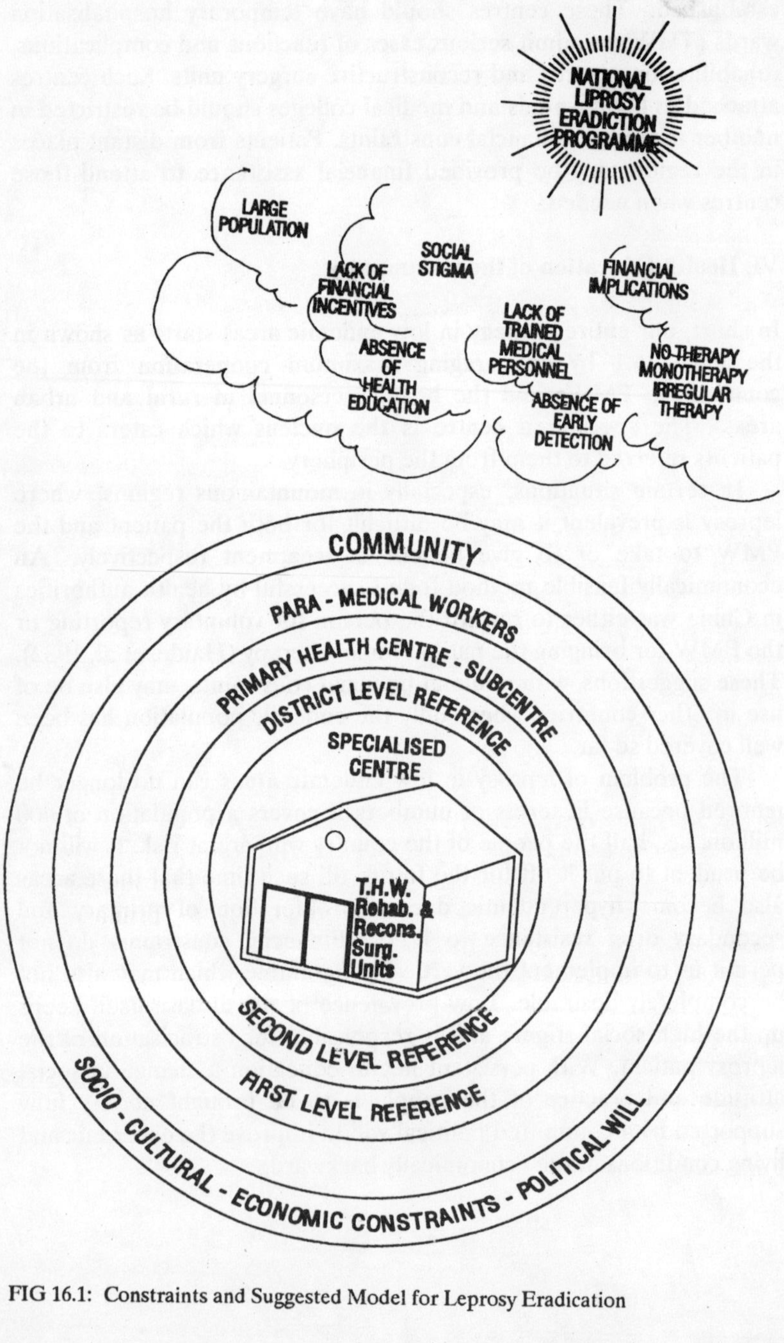

FIG 16.1: Constraints and Suggested Model for Leprosy Eradication

Community development programme, which was launched decades ago, needs to be meaningfully implemented at the level of primary health centres and sub-centres, because of late, WHO has also recommended the strengthening of primary health care (PHC) system in the context of leprosy. It has been defined as an integrated health system based on PHC approach and directing itself to equitable use of health resources, community participation and intersectoral cooperation.

The tasks at home, community, primary health centres, district hospital, regional and national levels need redefining in the process of evolving an integrated vertical-PHC approach. For this, training and re-training of medical and paramedical persons at the lower rung of the health set up is of utmost priority. This will ensure foolproof enforcement of MDT, monitoring of BI, and monthly follow up and surveillance nearer home.

By continuing medical education in the field of leprosy and in-service training of the health personnel in the matter of early detection of leprosy, day to day management, proper recording and reporting of the cases, referral of reactions and complications to regional specialised centres will become operative effectively.

The development of regional specialised centres with facilities for treatment, rehabilitation and reconstructive surgery under one roof with capacity for handling the complications of leprosy and maintaining a liaison with the periphery, i.e., Primary Health Centre and the community will ingrain confidence in the patients. Under prevailing social and economic conditions, an integrated vertical and PHC approach is the best solution with the necessary pre-implementation preparation.

The problem of low endemicity, as said earlier, is the problem of half the population in this country and even at the end of successful implementation in today's hyperendemic areas, it will persist and continue. To quote Noordeen, 'The most important technology is MDT which can reduce the global leprosy case load by 75 per cent in the next five to ten years. The latter phase, however, will not be easy to solve as they will consist of the breaking down of the old sub-clinical infections, difficult-to-reach cases, chronic defaulters and possibly some relapses, all occurring in a background of very low endemicity' (Noordeen, 1989).

REFERENCES

Bhatia, V.N., 1991, Management and Monitoring of Bacteriological Index *in, Report of Workshop on MDT of Leprosy in Low-endomic areas of India: An Evaluation*, Safdarjang Hospital, New Delhi, p 44-51.

Dharmshaktu, N.S.; Sharma, R.C.; Devarajan, L.; Mittal, B.N., 1987, A survey on population of multibacillary cases of leprosy in Himachal Pradesh, *Indian J Lepr*, 89, p 300-308.

Haide, M.; Gunyan, Y., 1989, Leprosy work in China, *Lep Rev*, 53, p 81-84.

Misra, R.S.; Ramesh, V., 1987, Leprosy in the Union Territory of Delhi, *Indian J Lepr*, 59, p 293-299.

Noordeen, S.K., 1989, Technology for leprosy control: Progress and prospects (Kellersberger Memorial Lecture 1988), *Ethiop Med J*, 27(3) July, p 161-180.

Pfau, R.; Haq, G., 1986, Leprosy in Pakistan, *Lep Rev*, 57, p 355-359.

Revankar, C.R.; Dudhalkar, B.; Raju, D.G.; Ganapati, R., 1986, Leprosy surveys in urban slums: Possibilities for epidemiological investigations, *Lep Rev*, 57, p 355-359.

Revankar, C.R.; Jha, S.S.; Dongre, V.V.; Deshpande, S.S.; Ganapati, R., 1982, Integration of leprosy into general health services in urban areas: A feasibility study, *Lep Rev*, 53, p 197-205.

17

BIOTECHNOLOGICAL AND IMMUNOLOGICAL APPROACHES IN LEPROSY CONTROL

RAMA MUKHERJEE

The rapid advancement in the biotechnology has made it possible to study the molecular basis of host-pathogen interaction, genetics of the pathogen and protective versus pathogenic host immune response. Research is also geared towards molecular dissection of the pathogen and development of highly purified molecules such as protein, lipids and sugar. It has been possible to develop antigens, antibodies and nucleic acid probes. Using the synthetic and recombinant techniques, it is feasible to design effective vaccines for the preventive and therapeutics of infectious diseases. Besides, the components of the pathogen which have been conventionally used for immunological interventions, other strategies to boost protective immune response or curtail adverse host immune response can now be used. Some of these strategies have already been applied in dissecting M. leprae and in leprosy control while others will be used in future. With the advent of good and reliable multidrug chemotherapy (WHO, 1982), the hope of curing leprosy and eradicating the disease from the face of earth has brightened. However, the experience of the past few years of the administration of the Multi-drug therapy (MDT), has revealed that although the disease is arrested, at the end of the therapy, multibacillary patients remain burdened with killed bacilli and the paucibacillary patients continue to harbour granulomatous lesions. Persistence of dead bacilli or granulomatous lesions puts the patients at high risk of lepra reactions or relapse. These patients slowly become bacteriologically negative over a period of time after release from therapy and the lesions too regress with time. The chemotherapy does not affect the immunological status of the patients suggesting thereby that multibacillary patients if re-exposed to M. leprae would not be able to mount protective immune response and remain susceptible to reinfection. Hence immunological intervention to boost the immunity, either prophylactically as a preventive measure or immunotherapeutically as an adjunct to chemotherapy for the rapid clearance of bacilli during the disease process, would have an important therapeutic role.

The immunological process of the disease is not yet understood. Vast research work conducted so far has thrown light on certain aspects of the pathogenesis of the disease, helped in understanding possible mechanisms underlying resistance and the possibility of developing newer and more effective vaccines against the disease.

What is clear now is that the causative agent M. leprae is an obligate intracellular parasite. It owes its virulence to its ability to survive within the macrophages and Schwann cells. Protective immune responses are of the cell-mediated type and serve to enhance the ability of the macrophages or Schwann cells to inhibit the replication or destroy the organsms *per se* (Kaufmann, 1990). In the cell-mediated immune reaction, T-lymphocytes play a major role. The most important T-cells are CD3+ T-cells which recognize antigenic peptides in the context of the products of the major histocompatibility complex (MHC) via a T-cell receptor composed of alpha and beta chain. These coventional T-lymphocytes can be further separated into two subsets which either express the CD8 molecule and recognize antigen in the context of Class I MHC molecules or CD4 molecule which recognize antigen in the context of Class II MHC molecules. There is significant data which suggest that CD4+ and CD8+ cell play a significant role in the control of mycobacterial infection. However, recently, besides T-cells expressing the beta receptor a second type of T-cell receptor composed of gamma-delta chain have been identified. These T-cells preferentially recognize mycobacterial components suggesting that they may have a role in intracellular bacterial infections. The functional activity of T-cells is to perform helper and killer functions. CD4+ cells carry out the function of activating macrophages as well as activation of effector cells by releasing sets of cytokines while the CD8+ cells with specificity for intracellular bacteria express cytolytic activity. The major advantage of target cell lysis would be the release of micro-organisms from host cells which by themselves are unable to restrict the growth of intracellular organisms. Thus the T-cell-mediated protection against intracellular bacteria is a concerted effort of helper T-cell of CD4+ phenotype-mediated macrophage activation and the target cell lysis by killer T-cell of CD8+ phenotype. Studies analysing the functional role of T-lymphocyte subsets on local application of recombinant interleukin-2 on reconstitution of CMI in the skin lesions in lepromatous leprosy patients further confirmed and emphasized the role of these two subset of T-cells. In addition, natural killer cells were also inducted. It is now becoming evident that if this concept is to be extended to an *in vivo* situation, for the cell-mediated immunity of protective nature to occur, multiple antigens will have to activate several subpopulation of T-cells. M. leprae specific unresponsiveness of the T cells is due to active suppression by the T-suppressor cells or suppressor factors or a combination of both (Bloom and Mehra, 1984).

Thus research is in progress in the identification and characterisation of individual components of mycobacteria involved in interaction with the immune system. It has come a long way making the possibility of developing new reagents for immuno-diagnostic tests and vaccine feasible.

Immunological Tools for Leprosy Control

Vaccine:	Based on live or killed bacillus	
	Synthetic peptides	
	Recombinant live :	Vaccinia virus
		Attenuated strain of *Salmonella typhi*
		M. w
Diagnostic reagents:	Recombinant antigen	
	Purified antigens	
	Polyclonal sera	
	Monoclonal antibodies	
Nucleic acid probes for early infection:	viability determination	
	monitoring chemotherapy	
Immunomodulators:	Interferon gamma	
	Interleukin - II	
	Soluble TNF receptors	
	Soluble IL-I receptors	

Vaccines

An appropriate or ideal vaccine has yet to be developed. The delay has been due to the inability to cultivate M. leprae *in vitro* in synthetic medium. It has partially been overcome by cultivating M. leprae in Armadillo (Kerchheimer and Storrs, 1971). Armadillo derived bacilli has facilitated biochemical, immunological and molecular characterisation of M. leprae. Mouse foot pad has been used for testing the potential vaccine candidates (Shepard, 1960). Vaccines currently on trial utilise either live or killed whole bacillus. The candidate vaccines BCG, M. w and ICRC have similar properties in the sense that these share several antigens with M. leprae involved in cell mediated immune functions, additionally also contain cross-reactive or non-cross reactive antigens which have the ability to break the tolerance of multibacillary patients, specially LL to M. leprae antigens.

BCG Alone or BCG+M. Leprae

Bacillus Calmette Guerin (BCG) imparts variable level of protection against leprosy, highest being in Uganda, and lowest in Burma (Myanmar) (Stone, et al, 1973; Kyaw Lwin, et al, 1985). In the mouse foot pad model, live BCG + killed M. leprae was able to confer protection against M. leprae infection (Shepard, 1976). Based on these observations, two large scale randomised controlled trials, each employing combined live BCG + killed M. leprae were initiated in Venezuela and Malawi with the support of IMLEP, WHO. The results of the first six years of trial in Venenzuela has revealed that addition of killed M. leprae had no additional advantage over immunization with BCG alone (Convit, et al, 1992). Such a result has been attributed to the natural decline in the prevalence and annual incidence of the disease and previous vaccination with BCG. The result of Malawi trial is awaited (Ponnighaus and Fine, 1986). However, encouraging and beneficial effects of combining BCG vaccine with chemotherapy has been reported (Convit, et al, 1982). Immunization with killed M. leprae + live BCG led to a faster recovery. Conversion of lepromin reactions was seen in 38 per cent of active leprosy, 63 per cent of inactive cases and a much higher conversion in the intermediate group of patients.

ICRC Bacillus

ICRC is an isolate cultivated from lepromatous nodules (Bapat, et al, 1958) and currently is under phase III clinical trials for both immunoprophylaxis and immunotherapy (Deo, et al, 1981, 1984). ICRC is reported to bring about persistent lepromin conversion in 53 per cent of lepromatous leprosy and 95 per cent of lepromin negative healthy contacts of patients in endemic areas. ICRC vaccine is being administered to volunteers in the general population. The immunoprophylactic efficacy of the vaccine is to be determined by its effect on the incidence of the disease.

Mycobacteria w

Mycobacterium w is a cultivable non-pathogenic Mycobacterium belonging to Runyon group IV (Saxena, et al, 1978). The results of phase II and phase III clinical trials for both immunotherapy and immunoprophylaxis conducted on multi-bacillary patients covering LL, BL and BB and leprosy patients contact are partly available (Talwar, et al, 1990). The vaccine is being administered to active multi-bacillary patients who are negative to Mitsuda lepromin. Their clinical, histopathological and bacteriological status were determined at the time of enrolment and then repeated after the administration of vaccine. Patients receive the MDT regimen recommended by WHO. Administration of the vaccine + MDT resulted in faster bacterial clearance from the lesions, clinical improvement and lepromin conversion from negativity to positivity leading to faster release from therapy of patients on immuno-chemotherapy as against patients receiving chemotherapy alone. The overall improvement was also evident in histopathology. There was evidence of immunological upgrading leading to complete disappearance of the dermal granuloma with a histological picture of a non-specific infiltration. The lepromin conversion was around 70-100 per cent in LL and BB respectively.

Gamma-interferon

Gamma-interferon is one of the principal cytokine secreted by activated lymphocytes which in turn activates the macrophages infected with M. leprae. This cytokine is either not produced or produced in low quantity in LL patients, therefore direct administration of gamma-IFN has been carried out in LL patients to boost the local CMI in the lesion. Gamma-IFN induced DTH reactions in the LL patients by 48 hr of injection. The macrophages in the granulomatous infiltrate were activated as evidenced by significant production of superoxide radicals and significant fall in bacterial load in the lesions (Kaplan, et al, 1989; Nath, et al, 1990).

Interleukin-2

The other approach adopted has been administration of *soluble T cell growth factors*. It is reported to induce good CMI in significant percentage of LL and BL patients leading to killing and clearance of M. leprae. There was evidence of macrophage activation, processing and presentation of antigens and induction of helper and cytotoxic T cells (Kaplan, et al, 1991). Many of the above-mentioned beneficial effects observed after administration of IL-2, or gama interferon are transient and do not lead to complete regression of the lesions necessitating the administration of these cytokines repeatedly. In addition, patients get some adverse side effects. A combination therapy of cytokines other than or in addition to IL-2 and IFN-gamma may have to be designed to be administered at the end of chemotherapy, i.e., before release from treatment, in order to facilitate rapid degradation and clearance of dead bacilli and aid in lessening the overall period of bacterial burden specially in LL cases with high BI. Such a combination is highly desirable while instituting wide usage of a short term course of highly effective combination of bactericidal drugs for as long as the bacilli are present and the risk of reaction and continuous slow tissue damage persists.

Other Cytokines/Soluble Receptors

The soluble mediators released by the mono-nuclear cells have both the physiological as well as patho-physiological role. The role of these mediators are now being examined by studying their production in the mono-nuclear granuloma infitrating cells, determination of the serum concentration in the various categories of leprosy and during lepra reaction. There is strong indication that the inflammatory cytokines, namely Tumor necrosis factor alpha (TNF-alpha), interleukin-1 beta (IL-1 beta) and Interleukin-6 (IL-6) may be playing important role in the pathological alterations at the site of the lesion, and, perhaps have a role in the of demyelination of nerve (Selmaj and Reine, 1988) and resorption of bone and cartilage (Thompson, et al, 1987). As a paradox to T cell anergy, the circulating inflammatory cytokines, i.e., TNF-alpha, IL-1 beta , IL-6 were high in the lepromatous group of patients and during Type I and Type II lepra reactions. Patients with high levels of circulating concentration of TNF-alpha went into repeated episodes of reactions.

Concomitant with the rise in serum concentrations, soluble TNF receptors I and II are also increased. These receptors have high affinity for TNF and their binding renders the serum TNF biologically inactive, thus limiting its pathological effect including nerve damage in leprosy. When TNF is complexed to its receptor, the active trimer form of TNF is established. Receptor and the complex TNF/soluble TNF (sTNF-R) may release free bioactive TNF. It is estimated that the sTNF-R should be around hundred fold higher than TNF in order to completely neutralise the bioactivity of the serum TNF. As the domain for the immunoreactivity and bioactivity are distinct, sTNF-R may be useful as a candidate therapeutic agent in persistant lepra reactions to mop up circulating TNF and the monoclonal antibody therapy will be of no consequence. Similarly, the antagonist to IL-1 beta or soluble IL-1 beta receptor could be used to arrest the ongoing tissue damage, in those patients where the reaction is associated with high serum concentration of bioactive IL-1 beta. Clinical trials with soluble receptor is a future prospect which has not yet been undertaken.

The measurement of cytokines in the serum of patients not responding to drug and exhibiting persistent reactions may also be significant. Our studies show that during type I and type II reactions, serum levels of TNF-alpha, IL-1 beta, and IL-6 were concomitantly elevated irrespective of the type of leprosy (LLs, BL, BB, BT), they initially belonged to the most frequent and highest level being that of TNF-alpha followed by IL-6 and then IL-1 beta (Parida, et al, 1992). The rise of TNF-alpha levels in these sera was associated with concurrent rise in serum levels of soluble receptors I and II. Patients with high serum levels of TNF-alpha and IL-1 beta were followed up for a period of 3-12 months. Hundred per cent of patients with serum TNF-alpha higher than 100 pg/ml and IL-beta higher than 200 pg/ml at initiation of the study went into repeated episodes of reaction within 1-3 months. These elevated levels have high prognostic value and measurement of serum TNF-alpha and IL-1 beta levels can be adopted in clinics in predicting the occurrence of lepra reaction. Soluble CD-23 and IL-2R were also frequently elevated in LL and reactional stage (Parida, et al, 1993). These cytokines also contribute towards the immunopathological process. The significance, however, remains to be determined.

Second Generation Vaccines

The current vaccines on trial are based on whole organisms. Several laboratories around the world are focusing their research on developing second generation subunit vaccine with better efficacy capable of inducing long term protective immune response, if not life long. The criteria for such candidate vaccines is gradually being evolved as we are beginning to understand the protective immune response. Any candidate antigens, whether protein and or lipid/sugars, should be able to induce immunity without causing any tissue damage or inducing persistent granuloma. Biochemical and molecular biological approaches have been adopted to purify the antigens. Several protein antigens of molecular weight ranging from 10 to 70 Kd molecular weight have been purified and their properties studied (Young, et al, 1985). Although several of these antigens stimulate T-cell mediated immune responses both *in vivo* and *in vitro*, these antigens failed to reverse the unresponsiveness to M. leprae antigens suggesting thereby that these antigens were not adequate as vaccines. The inability to trigger appropriate cell mediated immune response indicated additional need of adjuvants/carriers. This led to the approach of introducing genes coding for mycobacterial antigens into various potential vaccine vehicles, including vaccinia virus, BCG and Salmonella. In several experimental systems, vaccinia virus has been demonstrated to serve as a suitable carrier vehicle for recombinant proteins (Moss, 1985).

Its major advantage being the possibility of constructing a recombinant virus expressing multiple foreign genes. Thus it provides the possibility of constructing a recombinant virus expressing multiple M. leprae antigens with a gene coding for a lymphokine such as gamma interferon or IL-2. The other approach is the expression of M. leprae genes in other mycobacteria including BCG vaccine strains. It has been possible to introduce foreign DNA into mycobacteria using a recombinant shuttle plasmid (Bloom, et al, 1990; Jacobs, et al, 1987).

Investigations are continuing to improve recombinant DNA plasmids and develop methods that permit the insertion and expression of DNA into the mycobacterial genome. It is hoped that it will be possible to incorporate and stably express genes encoding M. leprae specific protective protein antigens identified in currently existing BCG vaccine strains.

A vaccine based on BCG has several attractive features including a "built-in" adjuvant effect, capability to confer certain degree of protection, low incidence of vaccine-induced complications, and a close taxonomic relationship of M. leprae.

Recently it has been possible to introduce genes in M. smegmatis as well as Mycobacterium w. Out of the three bacterial systems, expression of genes in M.w was the strongest (Bharati, et al, 1993). It is therefore possible that in future we would have a good live recombinant vaccine with higher immunogenicity and less delayed type of hypersensitivity effect.

Leprosy Vaccine: Future Prospects

Thus at present there are several vaccines based on whole organisms in clinical trial. Simultaneously research works at the laboratory level are on, to identify M. leprae specific protective antigens and their genes. Research is also directed towards finding a suitable vaccine vehicle for the insertion of the identified M. leprae genes of specific interest. Simultaneously the possibility of using purified protein antigens of M. leprae cell wall is also being explored (Vermani and Mahadevan, 1986). There is great hope that an ideal leprosy vaccine will be worked out in near future.

At the same time, problems related to leprosy vaccine development and trials have to be seriously considered, as leprosy poses some unique problems in relation to vaccine prospects (Noordeen, 1986). We need to know more about sub-clinical infection in order to discriminate between the infected and uninfected in the non-diseased population and to evaluate the role of the vaccine in the two groups. As regards the occurrence and pathogenesis of lepromatous leprosy and its immunological unresponsiveness, we do not know whether it represents a mechanism which can be interfered with a vaccine to the advantage of the infected person. Thirdly, there is apprehension that immunological upgrading of the population through the vaccine may result in an increased incidence of tuberculoid leprosy particularly in the initial period following vaccination. Role of environmental mycobacteria and M. tuberculosis in influencing the epidemiology of leprosy and possible interference in the efficacy of the vaccine, one way or the other needs to be understood. Therefore alongwith the development of vaccine, simultaneously research should be directed towards understanding the problems associated with vaccine trials as the implication of some of these problems are profound. If the vaccine is effective in uninfected and infected (frank and subclinical) individuals then it would not pose problems. But if the vaccine is effective only among the uninfected population and if M. leprae is highly infectious as is believed then the proportion of the population that will benefit will be so low that it will take several decades for vaccination to make impact on the disease situation in a highly endemic areas. Such a vaccine though may be good in low endemic situation, the number of persons to be vaccinated in order to prevent a case of leprosy will be quite large making the vaccine not effective from cost-benefit point of view. Finally the major difficulty with candidate leprosy vaccines is the length of time it would take to finally establish their efficacy for general human usage. During this period leprosy control programmes using early detection and multi-drug therapy would continue to play important role. The other important considerations are, good standard of vaccine without any batch to batch variation, good delivery system and subsequent follow-up.

An alternative strategy could also be thought of in the form of a vaccine for the prevention of nerve damage. Nerve damage leading to mutilation of the limbs is the main clinical manifestation responsible for stigma associated with leprosy. If a vaccine could be developed to prevent the entry of M. leprae into nerve cell or to arrest the M. leprae mediated nerve destruction then this organism could be reduced to relatively innocuous entity. Research is also being conducted in this direction (Mukherjee, R., et al, 1980; Mukherjee and Antia, 1985; Itty, et al, 1985 and Mukherjee and Antia, 1986).

Diagnostic Probes

Immunoassays Based on Antibody Detection

The earliest serological test, the FLA-ABS (Fluorescent leprosy antibody-absorption) test, was proposed in 1976 (Abe, et al, 1976). The test is based on detection of M. leprae antibodies in leprosy sera.

The percentage positivity for LL varied from 94.7 to 99.3 in comparison to 76.5 to 86.1 for TT (Bhardwaj, et al, 1981). However, the patient serum needs absorption with cardiolipin, lecithin and polysaccharide of tubercle bacilli, and sonicated suspension of BCG and *M. vaccae* to remove antibodies directed against cross-reactive antigens of M. leprae.

A number of enzyme immunoassays (EIAs) for immunodiagnosis of leprosy have been described. Of these the assays based on phenolic glycolipid I (PGL-I) are highly specific for leprosy. PGL-I (Cho, et al, 1983) is an antigen unique to M. leprae, and has a trisaccharide as the immunodeterminant. The terminal disaccharide and the monosaccharide residues of PGL-I have been chemically synthesized.

The assays based on PGL-I or synthetic sugar residues are quite sensitive for detection of active lepromatous patients with high bacillary road. In several independent studies with PGL-I, the percentage positivity for LL patients ranged from 58.4 to 100 in contrast to 35 to 57 for TT patients. Though the assay was highly specific for leprosy, a false positivity with tuberculosis sera has been reported.

The availability of M. leprae specific monoclonal antibodies (MoAbs) has provided a new thrust to the development of these immunoassays. In 1985 a serum antibody competitive test (SACT) using a MoAb (MLO4) directed against My2a determinant of M. leprae was reported (Sinha, et al, 1985). The assay is based on inhibition of binding of ^{125}I labelled MLO4 antibodies to M. leprae sonicate by antibodies in leprosy sera. The assay is highly specific for leprosy. Sera from normal healthy individuals, and patients with pulmonary tuberculosis or diseases such as cancer and auto-immune diseases were negative in the assay. Seropositivity was 100 per cent in multibacillary and 91 per cent in paucibacillary patients. False positivity with tuberculosis sera was 8.8 per cent.

By and large, most of the antibody based assays described above are quite sensitive for detection of multibacillary patients but the utility of these assays in diagnosis of paucibacillary leprosy is fairly low.

Immunoassays Based on Antigen Detection

Detection of M. leprae antigens in the clinical specimen (serum, urine, etc.) would be better indicators of infection. The detection of

PGL-I in serum and urine of LL and BL patients has been reported. The detection limit of the assay was about 50 ng PGL-I per ml of serum. It was observed that level of circulating antigen decreased shortly after initiation of therapy.

Nerve Antigen Based Assay

Most of the immunodiagnosic tests developed to detect the M. leprae antigen or antibodies are able to put into evidence only the LL form of the disease. An alternative approach is to develop a test that would measure the ongoing destruction of the nerve as a result of M. leprae infection. It would have a dual advantage of being a tool for the diagnosis of the disease as well as be a measure for the ongoing nerve damage or its arrest.

Using human nerve sonicate antigens a microtitre plate ELISA system to measure the antineural antibodies was developed by us. Sera belonging to LL, BL, BB, BT, TT and neuritis were screened. In this system, high titres of IgG class of antineural antibodies were detected in the sera in all categories of leprosy. The antibodies were also elevated in some of the contacts and early indeterminate forms of leprosy. In further studies this assay was refined and made highly specific. It was sensitive enough to pick up 95 per cent of the leprosy cases and was negative for tuberculosis, dermatological disorders and other autoimmune disorders such as systemic lupus erythematosus, Guillian-Barre syndrome and diabetic neuropathy. The assay was negative for normal healthy individuals (Mukherjee, et al, 1991).

Thus it is possible to put into evidence all the forms of leprosy if a combined serological test to detect M. leprae products or nerve products are used. Such a multi-test has yet to come out in the kit form for routine use in the hospital clinics or in the field.

The current and future research should be focused onto finding either a serological or nucleic acid probes that will determine the viability of the organism present in the lesion or diagnose very early indeterminate form of the disease. The test of the choice would be one which will discriminate healthy individuals from those who have subclinical infection. Therefore a battery of tests to determine the viability of the organism on one hand and to identify early infection on the other would aid the leprosy control programme considerably.

REFERENCES

Abe, M.; Izumi, S.; Satio, T.; and Mathur, S. K., 1976, Early diagnosis of leprosy by indirect immunofluorescence, *Lepr. India*, 48, p 272-276.

Bapat, C.V.; Ranadive, K.J.; Khanolkar, V.R., 1958, *In vitro* cultivation of an acid fast mycobacterium isolated from human lepromatous leprosy, *Ind. J. Pathol. Bacteriol*, 1, p 156.

Bhardwaj, V.P.; Ramu, G.; Desikan, K.V., 1981, Fluorescent leprosy antibody absorption FLA-ABS test for early diagnosis of leprosy, *Lepr. India.*, 53, p 518-524.

Bharati, J.; Mukherjee, R.; Young, D.B., 1993, Recombinant *Mycobacterium w* vaccine strain. (under publication).

Bloom, B.; Mehra, V., 1984, Immunological unresponsiveness in leprosy. *Immunol. Rev.,* 80, p 5-28.

Bloom, B.R.; Snapper, S.B.; Kieser, T.; Jacobs, W.R. Jr., 1990, Development of recombinant BCG vaccines, *Semin. Virol*, 2(1)

Cho, S.N.; Yanagihara, D.L.; Hunter, S.W.; Gilbert, R.H.; Brennan, P.J., 1983, Serological specificity of phenolic glycolipid I from *Mycobacterium leprae* and used in serodiagnosis of leprosy, *Infect. Immun.,* 41, p 1077-1083.

Convit, J., et al, 1982, Immunotherapy with a mixture of *Mycobacterium leprae* and BCG in different forms of leprosy and in Mitsuda negative contacts, *Int. J. Lepr.,* 50, p 415-424.

Convit, J., et al, 1983, Immunotherapy and immunoprophylaxis of leprosy, *Lepr. Rev.*, 51, p 475-605, special issue.

Convit, J., et al, 1992, Immunoprophylactic trial with combined *Mycobacterium leprae*/BCG vaccine against, leprosy, p preliminary results, *Lancet.,* 339, p 446-450.

Deo, M.G.; Bapat, C.V.; Chullawalla, R.G.; Bhakti, W. S., 1981, Potential anti-leprosy vaccine from killed ICRC, bacilli, p Clinico-pathological study. *Ind. J. Med. Res.,* 74, p 164-177.

Deo, M.G.; Bapat, C.V.; Bhalerao, V.; Chaturvedi, R.M.; Chulawalla, R.G.; Bhatki, W.S., 1984, Anti-leprosy potentials of the ICRC vaccine; A study in patients and healthy volunteers, *Int. J. Lepr.,* 51, p 540-549.

Itty, B.M.; Mukherjee, R.; Antia, N.H., 1985, Adherence of M. leprae to Schwann cells *in vitro*. *J. Med. Microbiol.*

Jacobs, W.R.; Tuckman, M.; Bloom, B.R., 1987, Introduction of foreign DNA into mycobacteria using a shuttle plasmid. *Nature,* 327, p 532-535.

Kaplan, G.; Mathur, N.K.; Job, C.K.; Nath, I.; Cohn, Z.A., 1989, Effects of multiple interferon gamma injection on the disposal of *Mycobacterium leprae Proc. Natl. Acad. Sci. U.S.A.,* 86, p 8076-8077.

Kaplan, G., et al, 1990, The reconstitution of cell mediated immunity in the cutaneous lesions of lepromatous leprosy by recombinant interleukin-3. *J. Exp. Med.,* 1691, p 893-907.

Kaufmann, S.H.E., 1990, Immunity to mycobacteria, *Curr. Opinion Immunol.,* 2, p 353.

Kerchheimer, W.F.; Storrs, E.E., 1971, Attempts to establish armadillo (Dasypus novemcinctus, Linn) as a model for the study of leprosy. 1. Report of lepromatoid leprosy in an experimentally infected armadillo, *Int. J. Lepr.,* 39, p 639-702.

Kyaw Lwin, et al, 1985, BCG vaccination of children against leprosy fourteen years findings of the controlled WHO trial in Burma, *Bull. WHO.,* 63, p 1069-1078.

Moss, B., 1985, Vaccinia virus expression, vector: A new tool for immunologists. *Imm. Today.,* 6, p 243-245.

Mukherjee, R.; Mahadevan, P.R.; Antia, N.H., 1980, Organised nerve culture II. DNA synthesis in Schwann cells in presence of M. leprae. *Int. J. Lepr.,* 48, p 189-192.

Mukherjee, R.; Antia, N.H., 1985, Adherence of M. leprae to Schwann cell *in vitro*. A specific phenomenon, *IRCS Med. Sci. Sept.,* 13, p 853-854.

Mukherjee, R.; Antia, N.H., 1986, Host parasite inter-relationship between M. leprae and Schwann cells *in vitro*. *Int. J. Lepr.* p 632-638.

Mukherjee, R.; Thomas, B.M.; Vemuri, N.; Talwar, G.P., 1990, Nerve antigen based serological tests for the diagnosis and prognosis of leprosy, *Trop. Med. Parasitol.,* 41, p 357-358.

Nath, I.; Laal, S.; Sivasai, K.S.R.; Tangri, S.; Murtuza, A.; Singh, S.; Wilfred, D.; Misra, R.S., 1990, Human immune response to recombinant interferon gamma and protein antigen LSR2, *Trop. Med. Parasitol.,* 41, p 324-325

Noorden, S.K., 1986, Epidemiological considerations in vaccine trials in leprosy, *Int. J. Lepr.,* 51, p 556-558.

Parida, S.K.; Grau, G.E.; Zaheer, S.A.; Mukherjee, R., 1992, Serum tumour necrosis factor and interleukin 1 in Leprosy and during lepra reactions, *Clin. Immunol. Immunopathol.,* 63(1), p 23-27.

Parida, S.K.; Grau, G.E.; Wallach, D.; Mukherjee, R., 1993, Soluble TNF receptors in serum of leprosy patients. (under publication).

Ponnighaus, J.M.; Fine, P.E.M., 1986, The Karonga Prevention trial with BCG, *Lepr. Rev.* 57, Suppl. 2, p 285-292.

Saxena, V.K.; Singh, U.S.; Singh, A.K., 1978, Bacteriological study of a rapidly growing strain of mycobacterium, *Lepr. India.,* 50, p 588.

Selmaj, K.W.; Reine, C.S., 1988, TNF mediates myelin and oligodendrocyte damage *in vitro*, *Ann. Neurol.*, 23, p 339-346.

Sinha, S.; Sengupta, U.; Ramu, G.; Ivanyi, J., 1985, Serological survey of leprosy and control subjects by monoclonal antibody based immunoassay, *Int. J. Lepr.,* 53, p 33-38.

Shepard, C.C., 1960, Experimental disease that follows the infection of human leprosy bacilli into foot pads of mice, *J. Exp. Med.,* 112, p 445-454.

Shepard, C.C., 1976, Vaccination of mice against M. leprae infection, *Int. J. Lepr.,* 44, p 222-226.

Stone, M.M.; Brown, J.A.; Kinnear, E.; Sutherland, I., 1973, The trial of BCG vaccination against leprosy in Uganda, *East. Afr. Bull.,* 2, p 15-24.

Talwar, G.P., et al, 1990, Immunotherapeutic effects of a vaccine based on a saprophytic, cultivable mycobacterium, *Mycobacterium w* in multibacillary leprosy patients, *Vaccine.,* 8, p 121-129.

Thomson, B.M.; Mundy, G.R.; Chambers, T.J., 1987, TNF alpha and beta induces osteoblastic cell to stimulate bone resorption. *J. Immunol.*, 138, p 775-779.

Vermani, M.; Mahadevan, P.R., 1988, A component of *Mycobacterium leprae* as immunomodulating agent-activation of macrophages to contain viability of M. leprae *in vivo* and *in vitro., in,* Proceedings of the IVth European Leprosy Symposium on Leprosy Research, Health Cooperation Papers, No. 7, p 153-161.

WHO, 1982, Chemotherapy of leprosy for control programmes. Report of WHO study group. Tech. Rep. Ser. 67, World Health Organisation, Geneva.

Young, R.A.; Mehra, V.; Swester, V.; Buchanan, T.; Clark-Curtiss, J.E.; Davis, R.W.; Bloom, B.R., 1985, Genes for the major protein antigens of the leprosy parasite *Mycobacterium leprae*, *Nature*, 316, p 450.

18

LEPROSY : Miles to Go

R.S. MISRA

Leprosy remains a major public health problem in 93 countries, of which 25 countries, with 10,000 or more registered cases, account for 95.2 per cent of the total registered cases in the world, and six of them (India, Brazil, Indonesia, Myanmar, Nigeria and Philippines) contribute 85.1 per cent, while India alone contributes 68 per cent of the global figure. After a steady increase in the number of registered cases between 1966 and 1985 (2.8 million in 1966 and 5.4 million in 1985), an increase of over 90 per cent over the 1966 figure, the trend had been towards decline (3.7 million in 1990) – a decrease of 31 per cent. While the increase in the registered cases in the initial phase (1966-1985) was due to increased awareness with regard to the disease and the need felt to combat it, the subsequent decline can be mainly attributed to the limited duration Multi-drug therapy (MDT) implementation and the resulting release from treatment of a significant number of patients.

The Leprosy Control activities are to be viewed in different regions of the world in the context of the Primary Health Care (PHC) set-up available in the country, socio-economic status of the populace, political set-up, stability and commitment to tackle the disease and MDT programme implementation. The gap between the registered and estimated leprosy cases is the most important parameter to assess the success of implementation of the Leprosy Control Programmes in a region. The level of health care facilities and economic viability are two other important factors in making available the most effective tool to control the disease, i.e., MDT. As an illustration it may be mentioned that, in India in spite of the commitment on the part of political leadership and availability of medical/paramedical personnel to a great extent, MDT could be implemented in less than half the districts of the country mainly due to financial constraints. The areas below 5/1000 prevalence remained out of the reach of the vertical programme, and the only treatment available in these regions was monotherapy, in spite of being fully aware of the high incidence of dapsone resistance.

MDT : Its Effect and Reach

MDT coverage in various world regions by late 1990, gives an idea about the reach of the effective line of treatment for leprosy, i.e., MDT.

Table 18.1 illustrates the fact that so far only 55.68 per cent of registered cases in the various regions of the world could be put on MDT, and this figure has remained dismally low in the African and American World regions at 18.37 and 23.75 per cent respectively. In African continent in the areas of high-endemicity, which are classified at level III A and level III B, the MDT coverage has remained 1/3rd or less. The Leprosy Control Programme in these areas had been either integrated with PHC set-up or combined with other specialised programmes, like tuberculosis, trypanosomiasis, schistosomiasis, immunisation, etc. (WHSQ, 1991).

TABLE 18.1: MDT Coverage by WHO Region, October 1990.

WHO Region	Registered Cases	Coverage %
Africa	482,669	18.37
America	301,704	23.75
South-East Asia	2,693,104	66.15
Europe	7,246	49.72
Eastern Mediterranean	99,913	38.67
Western Pacific	152,739	63.40
World	3,737,375	55.68

Source: Based on Document WHO/1991a.

MDT has succeeded in reducing the incidence of reactions in leprosy cases and has improved the treatment compliance by the limited duration for which the treatment is to be taken by the patients (Figs. 18.1 to 18.2). The fixed duration had also been responsible for discharging a back-log of large number of patients who were on monotherapy for decades without arrest of the disease process. This has further improved the health care delivery to patients attending leprosy treatment centres, and the better case-holding.

Due to financial and managerial constraints, viz., inadequacy of infrastructure to man the programme, the basic right of every leprosy patient to receive MDT, has not been fulfilled to a great measure so far. Any failure to contain the transmission of disease to the healthy population will be attributable to this factor in future. The other weak links in MDT areas had been (i) failure to ensure regular drug compliance, and (ii) adequate laboratory back-up to classify the patients as paucibacillary (PB) and multibacillary (MB) with a view to put them on respective regimen of treatment.

Therefore in future there should be only one line of treatment for all leprosy patients, wherever, they may live, with absolute goal of "MDT for all". This can be achieved in following two stages:

Stage I: by tackling all the accumulated known cases concentrating on 'proper case-holding'; and

Stage II: following it up, by establishing and maintaining "an effective case-finding as well as case-holding" (Ya Yuasa, 1991). Early diagnosis and effective MDT implementation is likely to reduce the disability incidence amongst the new leprosy patients, but old leprosy patients, continuing from monotherapy era, will keep on stigmatising the social outlook in areas where the stigma for leprosy is already high. These leprosy inflicted individuals, declared cured and bacilli free, need to be effectivly rehabilitated socially with the help of reconstructive surgery, providing them with adequate job opportunities, caring for them along with physically handicapped due to other causes, and not dealing with them in isolation. The last vestige of leprosy will be a deformed or disabled limb due to leprosy to be dealt with effectively by not only medical personnel but also with active cooperation of social scientists and community at large.

Role of Vaccines in Leprosy Control:

Vaccines can act as potentially inexpensive, safe, therapeutic/ prophylactic agents in leprosy control activities. The results of controlled trials with (BCG) vaccine have demonstrated varying levels of protection against leprosy — Uganda 80 per cent; Myanmar and Papua New Guinea 30 per cent; Chingleput, India 23 per cent, (ICMR, 1983). The first 5 years of follow-up of immunoprophylactic trial with combined Mycobacterium leprae/BCG vaccine has shown no substantially better protection than does BCG alone (Convit, et al, 1992). Immuno-therapeutic and immunoprophylactic trials with Mycobacterium w. and ICRC bacilli have been reported with varying degree of success in the matter of treatment (Figs. 18.3 to 18.5) and prophylaxis (Talwar, et al, 1990; Chaturvedi, et al, 1987; Kar, et al, in press). The work is going on towards the development of second-generation leprosy vaccines. The development of effective vaccine(s) against leprosy both for immunotherapeutic as well as immunoprophylactic purposes can serve as effective alternatives in control strategies in future.

Future Efforts in Leprosy Eradication

I. *Newer anti-leprosy drugs*

The work on testing the efficacy of newer drugs with bactericidal activities against M. leprae is in progress. They belong to three different classes : (i) fluoroquinolones, (ii) macrollides, and (iii) tetracyclines.

Ofloxacin, 400 mg daily and pefloxacin 800 mg daily, amongst the fluoroquinolones has demonstrated a high anti-leprosy activity. Twenty-two daily doses of pefloxacin or ofloxacin are reported to be capable of reducing by 99.99 per cent (or 4 $\log_{10}$) the number of viable M. leprae recovered from skin biopsies of leprosy patients. Multi-centric field trials in various countries are being undertaken by WHO, under exacting trial conditions during treatment phase and prolonged surveillance and follow-up. The outcome of the human trials will be watched with keen interest.

Among macrollides group clarithromycin (an-erythromycin derivative) and among tetracycline group minocycline have demonstrated a high anti-leprosy activity both in mouse-foot-pad system and humans, over a period variable from one to two months.

The potentiality of newer drugs in leprosy control programme is to be gauged to:

(a) Measure more precisely the anti-leprosy activities of each drug given alone or in combination with newer or standard anti-leprosy drugs, and

(b) Develop new drug regimens, curtailing the duration of the present regimen schedules and making them operationally more convenient.

II. *Preventing Disabilities in Leprosy*

The disability prevention can act as the greatest inducement in reducing the social stigma against the disease and thus giving boost to early case-detection and better treatment compliance. The future research is to be directed against the detection of 'silent neuritis', and effective and timely management of neuritis which may lead to deformities imminently.

III. *Care and Correction of Deformed/Disabled Limbs*

In this direction the programme priorities for disability prevention and rehabilitation need to be reoriented. In this context there is need to establish disability registers:

(a) to identify those with a high risk of having future disability,
(b) to identify those with disability, and
(c) to determine indicators for programme planning and evaluation.

There is need to integrate disability prevention and rehabilitation into general health care services and community based rehabilitation programme, not keeping the leprosy disabled in isolation and separate shelter. Caring of all the handicapped in one group will gradually wean away the stigma against leprosy.

IV. *Leprosy Control in Urban Set-up*

The leprosy control programme in the big cosmopolitan cities suffers from difficulties of early case-detection, regular monitoring for regular drug intake and contact tracing. This is due to long distances, shifting residential accommodation or employment places and loss of daily wages due to abstaining from work to collect the drugs at the Centre. The solution to these problems is to be sought on priority basis, by way of effective health-education (HE) to encourage passive case-reporting and establishment of a computerised registry for tracking the defaulters, and to ensuring that they are properly referred/transferred to other leprosy centres nearer their place of residence without disruption in treatment.

V. *Early Detection of Leprosy/Subclinical Infection*

The detection of leprosy in early stages is made out an easy job but the dermatologists and leprosy experts have found to their dismay that it is not to be considerd so easy. The diagnosis of 'indeterminate' leprosy, some times cannot be clinched by best of the investigative techniques available at. The hypopigmented macular lesions of face present difficult problems due to minimal loss of sensation in the lesion due to rich innervation in the area. Similarly, the early stages of lepromatous leprosy may only present with stuffiness in the nose and crusting in the nasal mucosa, making the patient least suspicious of the disease and at times testing the clinical acumen of the physician. The paramedical/medical personnel have to depend on evidence of leprosy in the close contacts to label such cases. There are no reliable laboratory tests available to suspect subclinical leprosy. There is need to develop new skin test antigens suitable for assessing such subclinical infections and estimating the epidemiological trends in infection.

VI. *Training of Medical/Paramedical Personnel and Programme Managers in Leprosy*

The training in leprosy in leprosy-endemic countries is by and large inadequate. Due to a large number of infective diseases prevalent in these areas along with nutritional and other deficiency disorders, leprosy has not received the adequate attention in the medical curriculum. A medical/paramedical person, unless and until trained beyond his normal training/curriculum, is totally incapable of dealing with the leprosy patients by himself. The 'Workshop on Training of Undergraduate Medical Students in Leprosy' sponsored by Gandhi Memorial Leprosy Foundation, Wardha, in collaboration with the Medical Council of India (MCI) pointed out the lacunae in the teaching of leprosy and recommended the need for strengthening the training programme from time to time (Appendix 18).

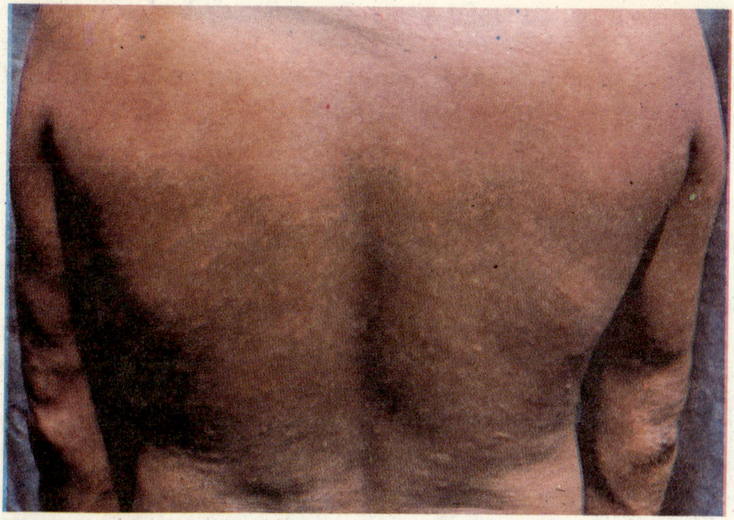

(1) Before MDT: B1 3.2, Histopathology LL

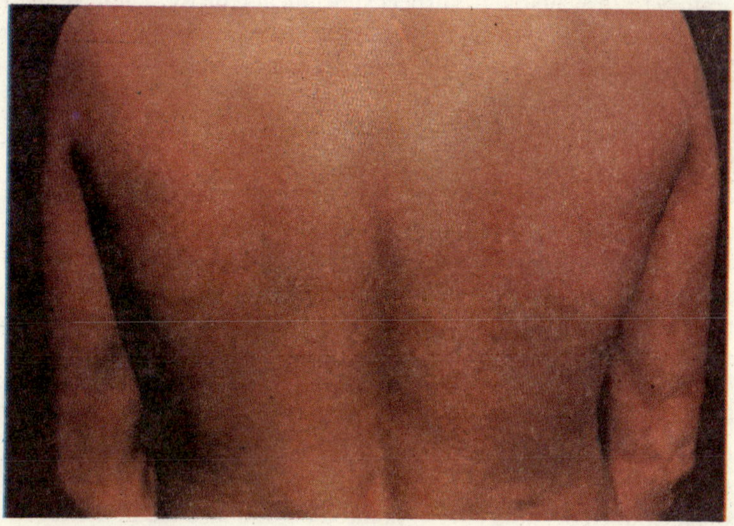

(2) After 2 Years of MDT : B1 1.5, Histopathology LL

FIG. 18.1: MDT in Lepromatous Leprosy

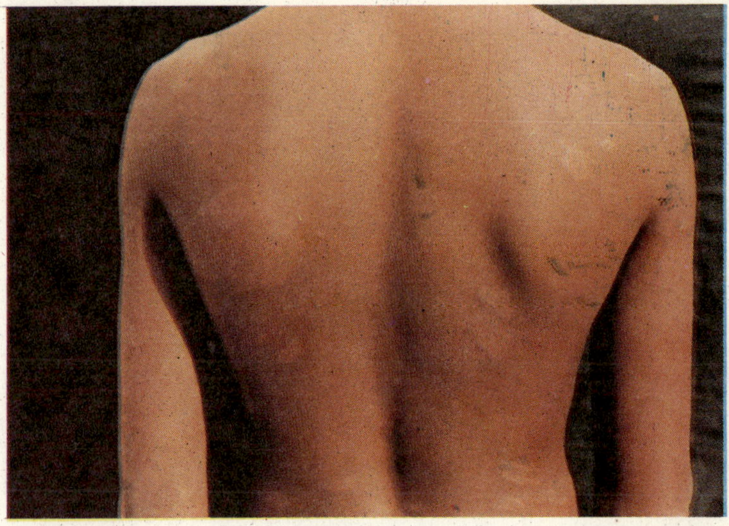

(3) Before MDT : B1 2.3, Histopathology BL

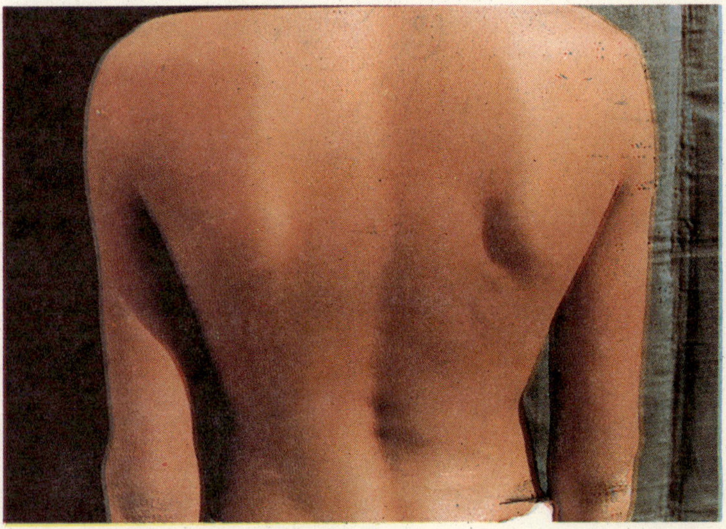

(4) After 2 Years of MDT : B1 0.16, Histopathology BL

FIG. 18.2: MDT in Borderline Infiltrates Leprosy

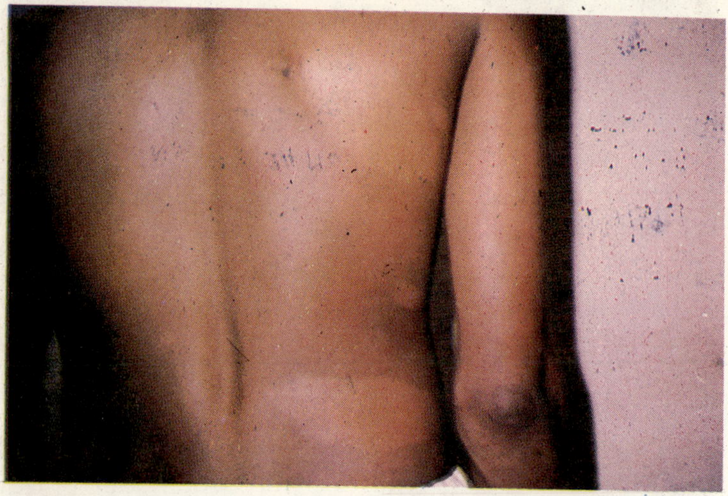

(5) Before Treatment : B1 0.33, Histopathology BT/BB

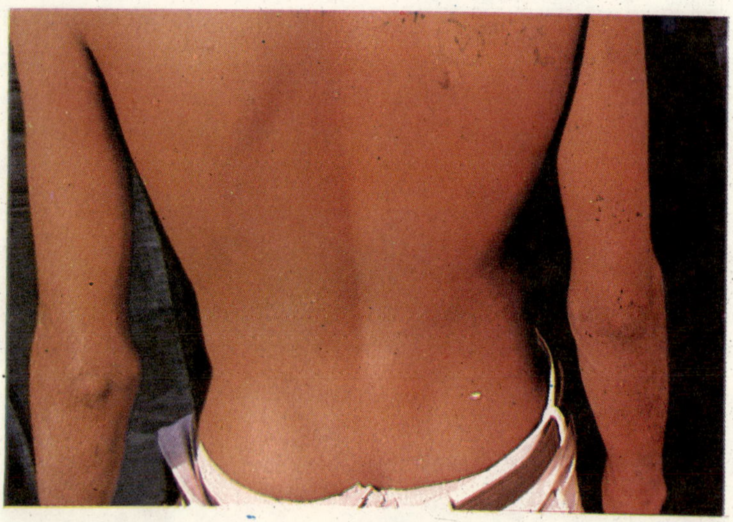

(6) After 6 Months of Treatment : B1 0, Histopathology — Non-specific Inflammation

FIG. 18.3: MDT with Mycobacterium W Vaccine in Borderline Macular Leprosy

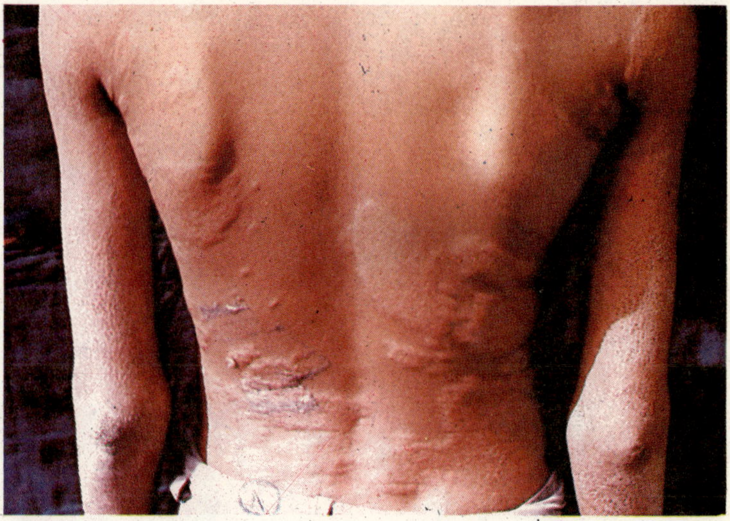

(7) Before Treatment BI 3.0, Histopathology BL

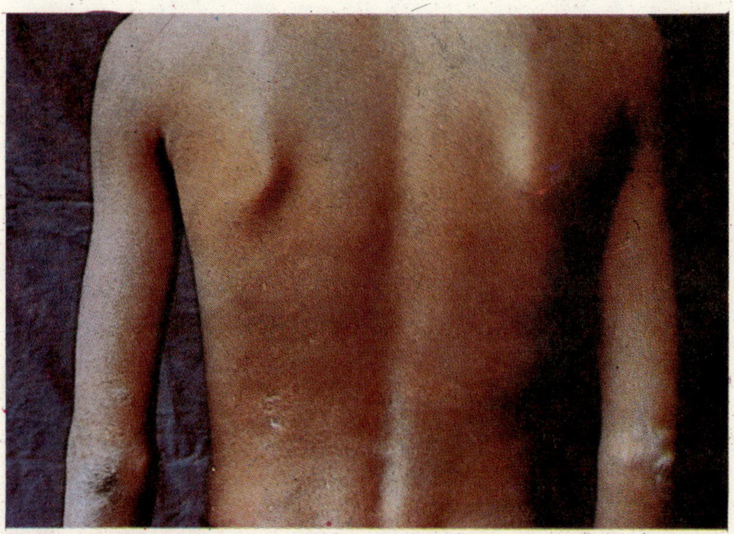

(8) After 12 Months of Treatment : BI 0.33, Histopathology BB

FIG. 18.4: MDT with Mycobacterium W Vaccine in Borderline infiltrated Leprosy

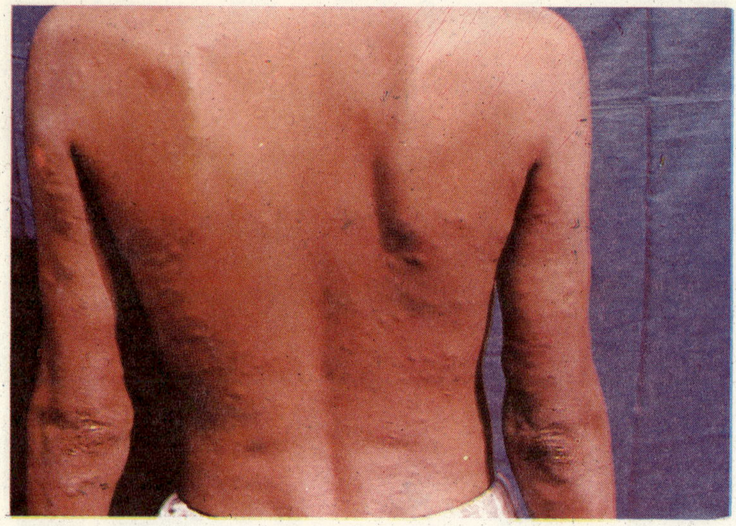

(9) Before Treatment : BI 4.0, Histopathology LL

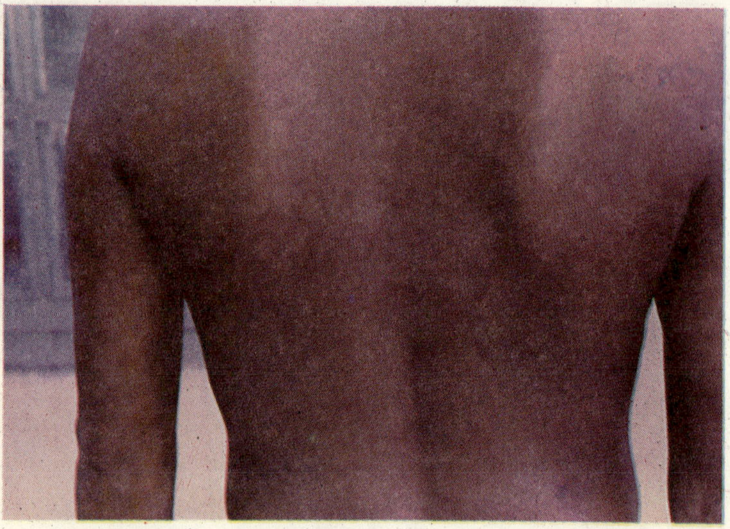

(10) After 24 months of treatment : BI 0.16, Histopathology: Non-specific Inflamation

FIG. 18.5: MDT with Mycobacterium W Vaccine in Lepromatous Leprosy

MCI organised a workshop of need-based curriculum for undergraduate medical education in August 1992 with the main aim of education in health sciences at undergraduate level to equip a doctor to function as a first contact physician who can provide basic health care to the community in its surroundings and handle emergency situations. Besides, he should be knowledgeable about the national policies, programmes and priorities directed towards the improvement of health situation in the country and be socially motivated and ethically committed to become a willing partner in the health delivery system of the country encompassing all aspects — preventive, curative and rehabilitative (Appendix 20). MCI appointed a committee for the purpose which prepared revised guidelines for medical curriculum in India during the decade of the 1990s. But the role of MCI is only conciliatory and it may take years to implement its recommendations in all the medical colleges in the country (Appendix 19).

WHO, in collaboration with the Royal Tropical Institute in Amsterdam (KIT), has developed training modules incorporating the know-how on organisation and management of leprosy control at the district level, integration of leprosy control activities with the general health service and the overall 'implementation of MDT" as the main component of control.

VII. *Health Education*

The health education activities in the community are to be updated from time to time, exploring all the communication media available to Health Educator in the area. This is to be done keeping in view the socio-cultural background of the community with an aim at dismantling the wrong notions, prejudices, etc., and directing it towards encouraging passive case-detection by early reporting and adhering to regular, full-time treatment as per programme requirement.

VIII. *Integration of Leprosy Control Programme with Primary Health Care (PHC) System*

WHO had been advocating the integration of leprosy control and care for leprosy patients into the PHC system to obtain optimal results with regard to WHO strategy for leprosy control based on early case finding, adequate treatment with MDT and health education (Appendix 22). The PHC approach is dependent on (i) equitable use of health resources, (ii) community participation, and (iii) intersectoral cooperation. Integration of leprosy control into the PHC system means that leprosy control activities will become the responsibility of decentralised, multipurpose and permanent health services which provide the community, including the leprosy patients, with integrated, comprehensive and continuous health care, within which a specialised leprosy component should be available for technical supervision, advice and referral.

The ill-planned process of integration, without taking into account the possible constraints and their rectification in advance, and without ensuring the smooth cooperation of the various participating units, can lead to difficulties which may be unsurmountable in future because of development of lack of credibility in the system. PHC integration will be dependent on the prevalence of the disease in the area, and the roles assigned to each level will have to be well-defined (Appendix 22). A proposed plan of action in this area has been discussed in Chapter 16 outlining the responsibilities of various levels of workers and the needed infrastructure for the purpose. The integration of leprosy programmes with the PHC system is to be tailored according to the prevelence of leprosy in the region and infrastructure available and their capability in the Primary Health Care set-up.

IX. *Coordination with Non-Governmental Organisations (NGOs)*

The governmental effort can be best channelised in the desired direction to achieve the goal of eradication of leprosy if the governmental agencies maintain a close liaison with and get full support of the community through a coordinated and preconceived efforts of various NGOs working the field. International Federation of Anti-leprosy Associations (ILEP) in cooperation with WHO seeks to use the contributions of the many hundreds of thousands of small donors in directly helping leprosy sufferers. The areas where NGOs can help to a great extent are in (i) training patients under MDT to take care of their hands, feet and eyes, (ii) establishing rehabilitation programme for all categories of disabled persons as per the community-based rehabilitation pattern, (iii) health education of the masses, and (iv) development of training modules for PMWs, and rehabilitation workers for the prevention of disability and for integrated rehabilitation.

The 44th World Health Assembly adopted a resolution on the

elimination of leprosy as a public health problem by the year 2000, underlying the effectiveness of the available treatment technology, i.e., MDT (Appendix 23). The experience of the past decade has demonstrated convincingly that it is possible to reduce the prevalence of registered cases up to 10-folds within a period of 5 years, provided MDT is applied to at least 80-90 per cent of registered cases (Noordeen 1991). But unfortunately this has not happened so far in the majority of regions and will be a tall order for the current decade as well, unless through health education, an awareness, towards recognition of early disease and breaking down the social barriers hindering patients self-reporting to the health services, is achieved.

MDT has succeeded as a chemotherapy, to kill the organisms harboured by the patient but not as a specific intervention in preventing nerve-damage and other complications leading to deformities – the most important stigmatising factor in leprosy. It is estimated that there are about 23 million individuals in the world who are disabled physically and socially as a result of past or present leprosy and that a significant number is likely to be added in the current decade resulting from late diagnosis and insufficient care. Thus, even if elimination of leprosy as a public health problem is attained, the problem of disability will persist. The only way this could be mitigated in future is by substantial improvements in the current technologies for prevention and management of nerve damage and deformities and their application in the field (Noordeen 1992).

'In the history of leprosy control, 1991 marks a turning point between the past and the future – a turning point that calls for a pause to take stock of what has been achieved and what remains to be done. If at this turning point in the history of leprosy, the momentum achieved in recent years is to be maintained, these needs and deficiencies must be addressed now. Never before have the means of eliminating leprosy been so readily available. Never before has there been such a global consensus over the possibility of using these means of achieve this aim. Now is merely not the time to slacken efforts but rather to prepare what could and should be the final chapter of the leprosy story' (WHO, 1991).

REFERENCES

Chaturvedi R.M., et al, 1987, Effects of ICRC Antileprosy Vaccine in Healthy Subjects, *Int J Lepr*, 55, p 657-666.

Convit, J., et al, 1991, Immunoprophylactic Trial with Combined Mycobacterium leprae/BCG Vaccine against Leprosy : Preliminary Results, *Lancet*, 339, p 446-450.

ICMR, 1983, *ICMR Bulletin* 13(9), p 89-91

Kar, H.K., et al, n.d., Induction of lepromin positivity by a candidate anti-leprosy vaccine "Mycobacterium to" in lepromin negative healthy contacts of multibacillary leprosy patients, *Ind J Lepr* (in press).

Noordeen, S.K., 1991, Elimination of leprosy as a public health problem, *Ind J Lepr, 63,* p 401-409.

Noordeen, S.K., 1992, Elimination of leprosy as a public health problem, *Lepr Rev, 63,* 1-4, editorial.

Talwar, G.P., et al, 1990, Immunotherapeutic effects of a vaccine based on a saprophytic cultivable mycobacterium, "Mycobacterium to" in multibacillary patients, *Vaccines*, 8, p 121-129.

WHO, 1991, Forty-fourth World Health Assembly, Resolution of the World Health Assembly, Agenda item 17.2 WHA 44.9, 1991 (Appendix 23).

WHO, 1991a, *Report of the First Meeting of the WHO Working Group on Leprosy Control,* WHO/CTD/LEP/91.4

WHO, 1991b, *Towards Elimination of Leprosy,* Leprosy Control Programme, World Health Organisation, Geneva, WHO/CTD/LEP/91.1.

WHSQ, 1991, *World Health Statistic Quarterly,* 44 (1), p 17.

Ya Yuasa, 1991, MDT for All : Target Oriented Leprosy Control, *Int J Lepr*, 59, p 624-638, Editorial.

APPENDIX 1

NLEP ORGANIGRAM : INFRASTRUCTURE FLOW

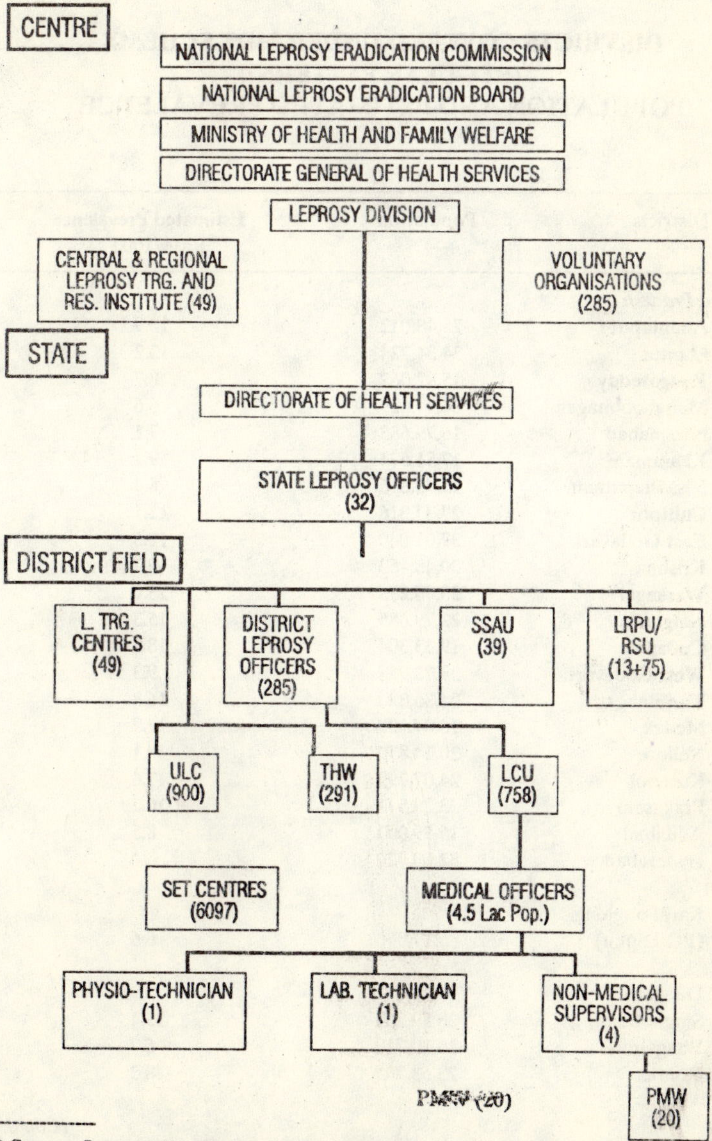

---

* Source: Leprosy Division, Directorate General of Health Services, Ministry of Health and Family Welfare, New Delhi.

APPENDIX 2

DISTRICTS COVERED UNDER MDT SCHEME (REGULAR PATTERN): POPULATION AND ESTIMATED PREVALENCE

State/Districts	Population	Estimated Prevalence Rate/1000
Andhra Pradesh		
1. Anantapur	25,48,012	12.9
2. Guntur	34,34,724	13.2
3. Rangareddy	15,82,062	8.7
4. Mehaboobnagar	24,44,619	6.6
5. Nizamabad	16,79,683	7.1
6. Khammam	17,51,574	9.1
7. Visakhapatnam	25,76,316	6.4
8. Chittoor	27,37,316	11.1
9. East Godavari	37,01,040	12.5
10. Krishna	30,48,463	9.7
11. Warangal	23,00,295	23.0
12. Nalgonda	22,79,685	15.3
13. Cudapah	19,33,304	18.5
14. West Godavari	28,73,958	9.3
15. Karimnagar	24,36,323	16.8
16. Medak	18,07,139	11.7
17. Nellore	20,14,879	17.1
18. Kurnool	24,07,299	17.6
19. Prakasam	23,29,571	10.2
20. Adilabad	16,39,003	8.5
21. Hyderabad	82,60,720	NA
Assam		
22. Karbi-anglong (PO Diphu)	5,17,000	6.6
Bihar		
23. Deogarh		
24. Singhbhum	28,59,260	15.4
25. Bhagalpur	26,10,719	6.7
26. Rohtas	23,63,705	18.2

(Contd.)

State/Districts	Population	Estimated Prevalence Rate/1000
Gujarat		
27. Dangs	1,12,664	6.2
28. Panchmahal (Godhra)	23,21,689	5.2
29. Surat	24,93,211	5.6
30. Bharuch	12,96,451	7.3
31. Valsad	17,74,136	6.9
Karnataka		
32. Bidar	9,95,691	8.00
33. Gulbarga	20,80,643	7.88
34. Raichur	17,83,822	10.52
35. Bijapur	24,01,782	5.87
36. Bellary	14,89,225	8.85
37. Mysore	25,95,900	6.21
Kerala		
38. Alleppey	18,94,805	6.56
39. Trichur	24,39,543	8.00
40. Trivandrum	25,96,112	6.00
41. Quilon	21,92,901	7.2
42. Palghat	20,44,399	10.0
Madhya Pradesh		
43. Durg	18,90,467	11.6
44. Rajnandgaon	11,67,501	13.5
45. Raigarh	14,43,197	16.0
46. Bilaspur	29,53,366	13.5
47. Bastar	18,42,854	5.2
48. Raipur	30,79,476	9.3
49. Bhind	9,73,816	9.1
50. Gwalior	11,07,879	13.1
51. Rewa	12,07,583	11.4
52. Ujjain	11,17,002	5.5
53. Sagar	13,23,132	5.4
Maharashtra		
54. Chandrapur	16,42,629	12.2
55. Nanded	20,24,364	10.1
56. Usmanabad	11,58,602	10.8
57. Yavatmal	19,82,252	8.1
58. Latur	14,45,294	10.8
59. Gadchiroli	7,38,138	12.2
60. Bhandara	20,36,415	7.1
61. Nagpur	31,07,097	7.2
62. Thane	42,44,486	7.5

(Contd.)

State/Districts	Population	Estimated Prevalence Rate/1000
63. Solapur	28,73,833	8.5
64. Satara	22,82,547	6.1
65. Parbhani	18,68,650	7.1
66. Raigad	16,61,643	6.5
67. Akola	20,80,926	6.3
68. Buldana	17,00,834	5.0
69. Beed	15,62,607	6.3
70. Bombay	100,81,753	6.0
Manipur		
71. Bishnupur	1,41,150	8.4
Nagaland		
72. Mon.	78,938	8.4
Orissa		
73. Puri	29,21,000	10.5
74. Cuttack	46,29,000	10.3
75. Dhenkanal	15,83,000	11.8
76. Mayurbhanj	15,82,000	12.8
77. Balasore	22,53,000	8.6
78. Sambalpur	22,81,000	16.1
79. Bolangir	14,59,000	14.5
80. Koraput	24,84,000	6.9
Tamil Nadu		
80. Chingalpattu	36,16,508	16.4
82. Salem	34,41,717	16.1
83. P.M.R. Sivaganga	9,72,576	17.5
84. Kamarajar	13,41,087	12.8
85. Ramanathapuram	10,21,774	10.9
86. Dharampuri	19,97,060	11.4
87. Thanjavur	40,63,545	13.8
88. Periyar	20,68,462	23.4
89. Q.E.M. Dindigul		
90. Madurai	30,17,172	14.3
91. South Arcot	42,01,869	16.9
92. Puddukottai	11,56,813	12.0
93. Tirchirapalli	36,12,320	10.7
94. Nellai Kota Bomman		
95. V.O. Chadamabarnar	13,50,874	9.9
96. Coimbatore	30,60,184	6.5
97. Nilgiris	6,30,169	—
98. Kanyakumari	14,23,399	9.0
99. Madras	32,76,622	12.0

(Contd.)

State/Districts	Population	Estimated Prevalence Rate/1000
Uttar Pradesh		
100. Varanasi	36,27,000	8.2
101. Barabanki	20,13,000	8.0
102. Dehra Dun	7,57,000	3.2
103. Faizabad	23,70,000	12.4
104. Sitapur	23,38,000	10.9
105. Kheri	19,63000	10.8
106. Kanpur (Urban)		
107. Kanpur (Dehat)	37,90,000	12.7
108. Uttar Kashi	1,91,000	8.9
109. Pilibhit	10,08,000	11.1
110. Bahraich	22,21,000	8.4
111. Deoria	—	—
112. Hardoi	22,94,000	10.1
113. Raebareilly	—	—
114. Azamgarh	—	—
115. Ballia	19,26,000	7.5
116. Gazipur	19,42,000	5.0
117. Mirzapur	20,34,000	5.2
West Bengal		
118. Bankura	26,64,542	12.1
119. Burdwan	54,47,744	10.0
120. Midnapore	75,65,416	10.0
121. Birbhum	23,51,519	12.0
Lakshadweep		
122. Lakshadweep	40,000	25.0
Pondicherry		
123. Pondicherry	4,44,417	13.0
124. Karaikal	1,20,010	8.0
125. Yanam	11,631	11.5

APPENDIX 3

DISTRICTS COVERED UNDER MODIFIED MDT SCHEME: POPULATION AND ESTIMATED PREVALENCE

(Population in Lakhs)

State/Districts	Population	Estimated Prevalence Rate/1000
Arunachal Pradesh		
1. Tirap	1,28,650	5.5
2. West Siang	74,164	9.5
3. East Siang	70,651	9.0
4. Towang	21,735	5.0
Bihar		
5. Dhanbad	21,04,381	15.9
6. Siwan	17,78,050	13.5
7. Patna	30,31,463	9.9
8. Aurangabad	12,36,528	5.5
9. Nawadah	10,99,067	8.86
10. Bhojpur	23,89,658	5.6
11. Purnia	35,92,637	5.8
12. Katihar	14,27,197	5.3
13. Muzaffarpur	23,53,283	5.85
14. Sitamarhi	19,29,827	7.05
15. Darbhanga	20,04,583	5.2
16. West Champaran	16,67,579	5.75
17. S. Parganas	37,07,160	5.8
Kerala		
18. Kasargoda	8,72,741	6.2
19. Ernakulam	25,35,294	5.0
20. Cannannore	19,30,726	5.0
21. Malapuram	24,02,701	8.0
22. Kozhikode	22,45,265	5.0
Madhya Pradesh		
23. Bhopal	8,39,739	11.2
24. Indore	14,09,473	13.5
25. Khandwa	11,53,580	8.9
26. Satna	11,53,387	9.6
27. Datia	3,11,893	7.5
28. Tikamgarh	7,36,981	5.4
29. Chhatarpur	8,86,660	6.6
30. Jabalpur	21,98,743	6.9
31. Balaghat	11,47,810	5.2

(*Contd.*)

State/Districts	Population	Estimated Population and Estimated Prevalence Rate/1000
32. Shahdol	13,45,125	5.6
33. Surguja	16,33,476	5.3
Manipur		
34. Tamonglug	62,289	7.0
35. Chandel	56,444	7.2
36. Phulbani	7,17,000	8.7
Orissa		
37. Sundergarh	13,38,000	10.5
38. Kalahandi	13,39,000	5.0
39. Keonjhar	11,14,000	8.8
A & N Islands		
40. Andaman	1,58,000	5.6
Nicobar	0,31,000	1.7
Sikkim		
41. East District	1,38,746	8.6
42. South District	75,545	7.9
43. Gorakhpur	37,96,000	5.9
Uttar Pradesh		
44. Lucknow	20,17,000	5.7
45. Unnao	18,27,000	6.8
46. Rampur	11.77	5.4
47. Badaun	19,69,000	5.5
48. Shahjahanpur	16,49,000	7.9
49. Etawah	17,49,000	5.7
50. Fatehpur	15,73,000	9.6
51. Banda	15,36,000	5.6
52. Hamirpur	11,94,000	7.7
53. Jalaun	9,88,000	7.1
54. Basti	35,77,000	6.0
55. Gonda	20,38,000	5.9
56. Bareilly	22,65,000	7.2
West Bengal		
57. Cooch Bihar	19,87,782	5.0
58. Howrah	33,28,817	5.0
59. Hooghly	39,91,297	5.0
60. Jalpaiguri	24,85,054	7.0
61. Malda	22,79,758	6.0
62. 24 Parganas (S)	50,19,010	5.0
63. Nadia	33,25,891	6.0
64. 24 Parganas (N)	66,16,806	5.0
65. W. Dinajpur	26,98,349	6.0
66. Murshidabad	41,48,216	6.0

APPENDIX 4

OLD MDT DISTRICTS PROPOSED TO BE INTEGRATED WITH GENERAL HEALTH CARE

Sl. No.	State/Districts	Sl. No.	State/Districts
	Andhra Pradesh		*Orissa*
1.	Srikakulam	8.	Ganjam
2.	Vijayanagram		
			Tamil Nadu
	Gujarat	9.	Ambadkar District
3.	Baroda	10.	T.S. District
	Karnataka		*West Bengal*
4.	Belgaum	11.	Purulia
5.	Dharwad		
	Maharashtra		
6.	Amravati		
7.	Wardha		

APPENDIX 5

LOW ENDEMIC DISTRICTS COVERED UNDER MDT

State/District	State/District
Gujarat	*Maharashtra*
1. Kheda	24. Ratnagiri
2. Ahmedabad	25. Dhule
3. Gandhi Nagar	26. Ahmednagar
4. Junagarh	27. Pune
5. Sabarkantha	*Manipur*
6. Banaskantha	28. Thoubal
7. Mehsana	29. Imphal
8. Surendarnagar	*Meghalaya*
9. Bhavnagar	30. W. Garohills
10. Amreli	31. E. Khasihills
11. Jamnagar	*Mizoram*
12. Kutch	32. Lunglai
13. Rajkot	33. Chimtuipud
Haryana	34. Aizawal
14. Faridabad	*Punjab*
15. Karnal	35. Ropar
16. Rohtak	36. Jalandhar
Himachal Pradesh	37. Ludhiana
17. Shimla	*Rajasthan*
18. Sirmour	38. Alwar
19. Solan	*Tripura*
Karnataka	39. N. Tripura
20. Kolar	40. S. Tripura
21. U. Kannada	41. W. Tripura
22. D. Kannada	*Uttar Pradesh*
23. Mandya	42. Saharanpur

APPENDIX 6

NLEP MULTIBACILLARY/PAUCIBACILLARY LEPROSY PATIENT CARD*

1. **Identification**

1.1 State/UT

1.2 District

1.3 L C U

1.4 Centre and Circuit

1.5 Village

1.6 MDT No.

1.7 Patient's old/cross reference No.

1.8 Name

1.9 Father/Husband's Name

1.10 Year of birth

1.11 Sex: M/F

1.12 Status: Married/Unmarried/Widow/Divorced

1.13 Address

1.14 Occupation

1.15 Caste

---

2. **Type of Leprosy**

2.1 PB (I: TT; BT; N)
MB (BB, BL, LL, N?L, BI Positive)

2.2 Duration of disease:
Month......... Year..........

2.3 Date of detection: Month......... Year..........

2.4 Date of registration Month......... Year..........

2.5 Mode of detection:
General Survey/Contact Survey/School Survey/Referred by PHC/Others.

2.6 Nature and Duration of Treatment: Years
DAPSONE, MDT—PB, MDT—MB

(Contd.)

---

* Source: *Leprosy, National Leprosy Eradication Programme in India, 1987,* Leprosy Division, Directorate General of Health Services, Ministry of Health and Family Welfare, Nirman Bhavan, New Delhi.

3. **Screening (By whom)** Date: Month Year

(A) *History of*:		(B) *Clinical Examination for*:	
1. Jaundice	Yes/No	1. Jaundice/Enlarged and/or tender liver	Yes/No
Alcoholism	Yes/No		
2. Chronic Cough	Yes/No	2. Abnormal Chest Findings	Yes/No
Haemoptysis	Yes/No		
3. Oedema of feet/	Yes/No	3. Enlarged Lymph nodes	Yes/No
face	Yes/No		
4. Pregnancy	Yes/No		

(C) *Laboratory Tests* 1. Urine 2 Hb. 3. Sputum:

---

4. **Assessment of Medical Officer**

1. Pulmonary Tuberculosis	Yes/No	2. Hepatitis	Yes/No
3. Anaemia	Yes/No	4. Renal Complications	Yes/No
5. Intercurrent Infections	Yes/No	6. Pregnancy	Yes/No
7. Socio-economic rehabilitation needed	Yes/No		

Comments : Is the patient eligible for MDT? If no, give reason.

Signature of M.O.

Date: (Name in Capitals)

RECORDING OF CLINICAL DATA

*See coding key

	Initial		6 months		1 Yr.		2 Yrs.		3 Yrs.		4 Yrs.		5 Yrs.	
	Old	New	Old	New	Old	New	Old	New	Old	New	Old	New	Old	New
1. Skin Lesions (a)Location (give No)														
(b)Number														
(C)Ap-Fl/Ra Ery/Hy														
(d)Dis-Sym/ Asym														
(e)Inf-N/Mi/MO/ Sev														
(f)Mar-V-ill def/ WD														
(g)Sur-Dry/SC/ Sh														
(h)Nod-N/F/M														
(i)Anaes-NA/PA/ CA														
2.Ear Lobes-N/Th/ Nod/Wr														
3.Eyes: (a) Cor An Pr														
(b) Pa/Red/Wat														
(c) Bl Vis/Lo														
(d) Cor Ul/Ir/Ircy														

Note: *See* Explanation of coding for clinical examination.

5. AT SCREENING–Date:

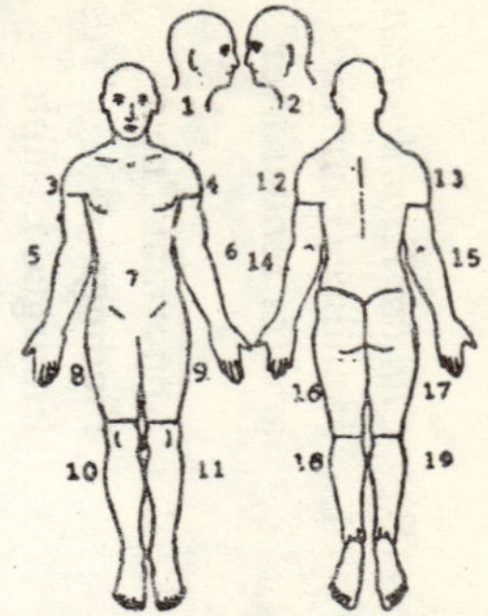

SUBSEQUENT CLINICAL OBSERVATIONS–Date:

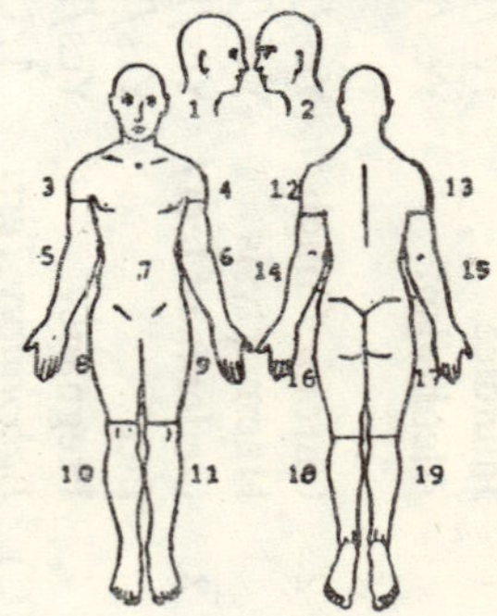

6.* NERVE INVOLVEMENT — Yes/No. If Yes:

Date Side	Initial		J		2		3		4		5	
	Lt.	Rt.	Lt.	Rt.	Lt.	Rt.	Lt.	Rt.	Lt.	Rt.	Lt.	Rt.
(a) Ulnar												
(b) Median												
(c) Radial												
(d) Lateral Popliteal												
(e) Posterior Tibial (f) Others												
7.* DISEASE STATUS												
8.* DEFORMITY/ DISABILITY:												
(a) Anaesthesia: (1) Polantar (2) Palmar												
(b) 7th Cr. N—Lagophthalmos												
(c) Ulnar-Claw hand-2 fingers												
(d) Median-claw hand 4 fingers												
(e) Radial-Wrist drop												
(f) Lat. Popliteal foot-drop												
(g) Posterior tibial claw toes												
(h) Plantar ulcer												

6.*Nerves: Normal — N, Enlarged — E, Tender — T, 7. * Disease Status (Clinical & Bacteriological, Active — A, Inactive — IA, 8.* Deformity, Disability: Present — P, Absent — A.

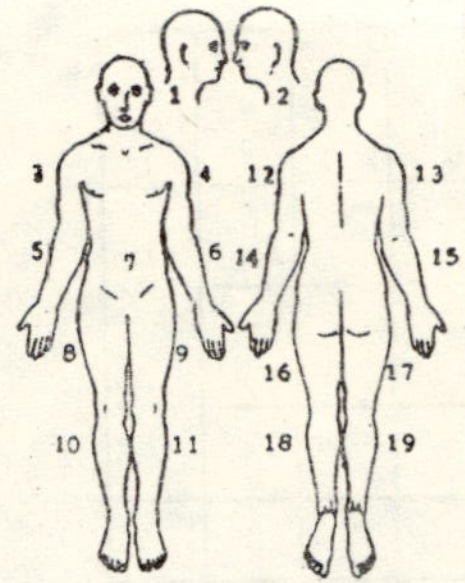

CLINICAL OBSERVATIONS:
At Release from Treatment Date:

4. Bacteriological Examination

Year	Date taken	Date exam	Results by site				
			1	2	3	4	5
Initial							
1							
2							
3							
4							
5							

5. Drug compliance tests

Date			
Method — Tablet count (TC/Spot test (SP) result			

Correct — C, Wrong — W, Positive — P, Negative — N.

Treatment Record

A. *Intensive Phase (For MB cases only) total days taken* Date started

Day	1	2	3	4	5	6	7	8	9	10	11	12	13	14
Rifampicin														
Dapsone														
Clofazimine														
Initials/MO/NMS														

If Intensive Phase not given, reason:

B. *Pulse Treatment* Date started

1st Yr.—Month	1	2	3	4	5	6	7	8	9	10	11	12	13
Rifampicin													
Dapsone													
Clofazimine													
Reactions 1, 2, N													
Initials of MO/NMS													
2nd Yr.—Month													
Rifampicin													
Dapsone													
Clofazimine													
Reactions 1, 2, N													
Initials of MO/NMS													
3rd Yr.—Month													
Rifampicin													
Dapsone													
Clofazimine													
Reactions 1, 2, N													
Initials of MO/NMS													

Deteriorating during Treatment/Evidence of Relapse:
Date Action taken:
If Treatment Discontinued, Reason Date:
(a) Refused, (b) Left project Area/District, (c) Side effects/Adverse reactions, (d) Died
Action taken if (a) or (b) or (c)

MULTIBACILLARY/PAUCIBACILLARY LEPROSY PATIENTS CARD CODING KEY

Explanation of Patient Card

The assessments cover initial examination at the time of screening and five subsequent examinations.

1. Identification
2. Types of Leprosy

Self-explanatory.

2.1 *Classification*

Patients should be classified as PB or MB as per the guidelines on the NLEP (1985). Any patient who was previously skin smear positive or now positive should be treated as Multibacillary. After recording the signs, symptoms, etc., the disease should be classified preferably under consensus classification of IAL.

2.2 Duration of disease — estimated date of onset of the disease.

2.3 Date of detection — Date of detection of leprosy by the PMW.

2.4 Date of Registration — Date when patient was put on therapy, monotherapy or MDT.

2.5 Mode of detection.

2.6 Nature and Duration of treatment: Indicate total duration of earlier treatment and as to what treatment was given.

3. Screening by whom

Persons's name should be clearly written with date.

3.1 History of recent jaundice and/or chronic alcoholism, to rule out liver dysfunction.

3.2 History of chronic cough/haemoptysis/enlarged lymph nodes to rule out pulmonary tuberculosis.

3.3 Oedema feet — to rule out any kidney involvement.

3.4 Pregnancy — MDT should not be initiated during 1st trimester if detected.

3.5 Indicate if any laboratory investigation done.

4. Assessment of Medical Officer

The reason for this assessment is three fold:

4.1 Confirm diagnosis and classification.

4.2 Assess eligibility for MDT and rule out contra-indication prior to start of MDT.

4.3 Make a careful clinical record of the patients so that subsequent progress of the disease can be monitored.

Assess socio-economic rehabilitation needs of the patients in consultation with the PMW/NMS.

Eligibility for MDT — Certification that patient is eligible for MDT with no contra-indication.

Any comments.

5. Provision for three body chartings is there in the record. One at the time of screening the other during therapy, if any evidence of deterioration/need for change in therapy from PB to MB, etc., and the last at time of release from treatment.

Explanation for coding for clinical examination

Initial — is the assessment at time of screening, followed by assessments at 6 months and 1-5 years follow-up.

Old — refers to old lesions present at screening.

New — If any new lesions develop subsequently, the short coding above should be filled where applicable. If the appearance is flat then put Fl in the concerned column. If multiple lesion is flat and raised put Fl/Ra.

1. (a) Location give numbers as in body chart.
   (b) Numbers = 1, 2—4, 5—9, $\geq$ 10.

(c) App = Appearance; Fl = Flat, Ra = Raised, Ery = Erythematous
(d) Dis = Distribution; Sym = Symmetrica; Asym = Asymmetrical
(e) Inf = Infiltration; N = None; Ml = mild; MO = Moderate; Ser = Severe
(f) Mar = Margins; V = Vague/ ill def = ill defined; WD = Well defined
(g) Sur = Surface; Dry, SL = Scaly, Sh = Shiny
(h) Nod—Nodules; N—None; F—Few; M—Many
(i) Anaes—Anaesthetic, NA—Not anaesthetic, PA—Partially anaesthetic; CA—Completely anaesthetic

2. Ear lobes—N—Normal, Th—Thickened, Nod—Nodular, Wr—Wrinkled.

3. Eyes—
(a) Cor An Pr—Corneal Anaesthesia Present.
(b) Pa—Pain, Red—Redness, Wat-Watering.
(c) Bl Vis—Blurred Vision, Lo—Loss of vision
(d) Cor Ul—Corneal Ulser, Ir—Iritis, Ircy—Iridocyclitis.

4. *Bacteriological (BI) Examination*: The Bl should be recorded in the Ridley Scale (0–6+). The sites once taken should be consistently the same. The usual sites being (1) At right ear lobe (2) Right eye brow (3) Chin (4) Right buttock (in women right thigh) (5) Any special site.

5. *Drug Compliance*: should be checked periodically by tablet counts or simple urine spot tests wherever possible.

6. *Nerve Involvement*: Involvement ofthe major trunk nerves as indicated Special attention should be given to examine the nerves and muscles supplied by them for evidence of early paresis/paralysis.

7. *Disease Status:* Indicate whether patient is Active or Inactive, clinically and bacteriologically.

8. *Deformity/Disability:* The assessment should be done with the following in mind:

1. Identifying patients who can benefit from surgery.
2. Accurately recording nerve dysfunction so that progress can be monitored over the years.

3. Identifying patients at risk of injury (grade-1).
(i) Patients needing surgical correction should be identified and referred for treatment.
(ii) The WHO deformity grade is as follows:
Grade 0 — No anaesthesia no deformity.
Grade 1 — Anaesthesia
Grade 2 — Correctable deformity
(mobile claw hand etc.)

9. *Treatment Records:* For a 3 year period is provided for. A (✓) tick indicates that the patient attended. For pulse therapy the recommended duration is at lest 24 months. If clinics are held once every calender month say Jan/Feb. etc. then there will be 12 entries for 1 year. If clinics arre held once every 4 weeks, there will be 13 entries every year or 26 for 2 years.

If reactions are present, indicate whether type—1 or type—2, N—None.

10. If there is any deterioriation during therapy or evidence of relapse after cessation write what action taken.

11. If treatment discontinued, give reason. Special attention should be paid to cessation of therapy due to side effects of drugs or complication of therapy.

APPENDIX 7

KEY TO BODY CHARTING OF LEPROSY PATEINTS*

2

Definitions

Macule : A skin lesion flush with the surface of the skin.
Papule : A thickened lesion in the skin of a size below one cm. in diameter.
Nodule : Similar to a papule but larger than one cm. in diameter.
Plaque : A patch in the skin with its entire surface raised above the surface of the skin.

1. Ill-defined hypopigmented macule: 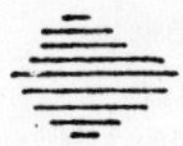
2. Infiltration: 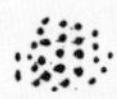
3. Resolving macule: 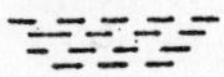
4. Partial sensory loss: 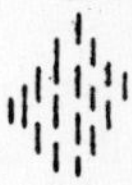
5. Anaesthesia: 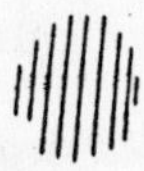
6. Well defined hypopigmented macule with anaesthesia: 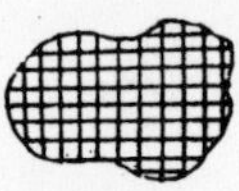
7. Well defined patch with anaesthesia: 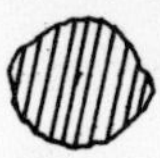

---

2. * Source: *Leprosy: National Eradication Leprosy Programme in India 1987*, Leprosy Division, Directorate General of Health Services, Ministry of Health and Family Welfare, New Delhi.

8. Well defined macule: 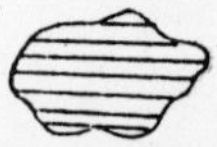

9. Well defined patch, anaesthetic with central healing: 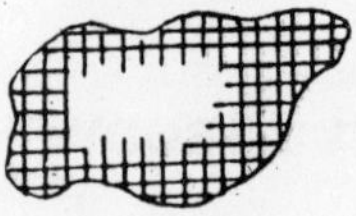

10. Well defined anaesthetic patch with infiltrated borders which are raised: 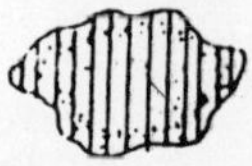

11. Pebbly appearance: 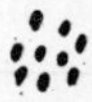

12. Patch with one margin ill-defined macular: 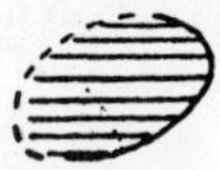

13. Nodules: 

14. Nerves which are thickened: 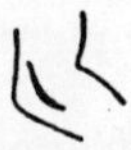

15. Loss of digits: Claw fingers: 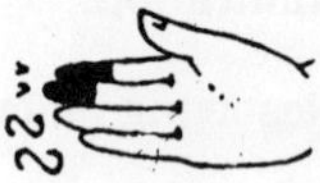

16. Gynecomastia: Gyneothelia: 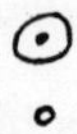

17. Foot drop wrist drop against area: 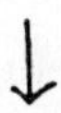

18. Ulcer on sole of foot: Ulcer scar: 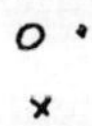

19. Collapse nose: 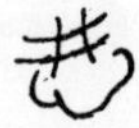

20. Loss of eyebrows: 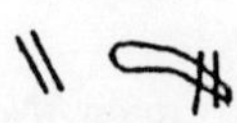

APPENDIX 8

ORIENTATION TRAINING SCHEDULE FOR VARIOUS CATEGORIES OF WORKERS FOR MODIFIED MDT IMPLEMENTATION

Sl. No.	Name of the category	Duration of orientation training	Place of orientation training	By whom
1.	RMPs, Village leaders Opinion leaders, NSS students, Youth Clubs, Mahila mandals, Angan-Wadi Workers.	One day	To suit local conveniences	MO of PHC with the help of DLO & staff
2.	DPRO, TV, AIR, Central FP, Film Unit, etc.	One day	District headquarters	CDMO & DLO
3.	School teachers	One day preferably on central class day	School where central class is held	MO, PHC/ NMS
4.	Vol. Organs., Lions Club, Rotary, etc.	One day	District headquarters	CDMO & DLO
5.	Teaching staff of Medl. Colleges, Deptt. of Dermatology, Neurology, Preventive Medicines, etc.	One day	To suit local conveniences	SLO
6.	Industrial establishments, public undertakings etc.	One day	To suit local conveniences	DLO & MO
7.	Health Guides	One day (on monthly) meeting day	PHC headquarters	MO, PHC, NMS

ORIENTATION TRAINING SCHEDULE FOR PRIMARY HEALTH CARE STAFF FOR IMPLEMENTATION OF MODIFIED MDT

Modified MDT is to be implemented by the Primary Health Care staff for the first time in the endemic districts. The role of the NLEP vertical staff in these districts is limited to provide technical support/guidance. Hence, it is very essential to give adequate and appropriate orientation to Primary Health Care staff to enable effective implementation of MDT. It is also necessary to keep in view their existing work load while entrusting additional functions under MDT. Keeping these facts in view the following schedule is worked out:

Sl. No.	Name of the category	Duration	Place of trg.	By whom	Remarks
1.	CDMOs, DLOs.	One day	Distt. Hqrs.	Central Training Team	
2.	MOs, PHCs/SHCs.	4 days	Distt. Hqrs.	Central Training Team with the help of CDMO and DLO who had one day discussion	
3.	MPW Supervisors and MPWs.	3 days	PHC Hqrs.	DLO, MO, PHC and NMS	
4.	Available NLEP	One day	Distt. Hqrs.	CDMO and DLO	

STATEWISE LEPROSY PROFILE AND PROGRESS OF NLEP IN INDIA, 1991

Sl. No.	Name of State	Popul. 1991 (lakhs)	Estd. Prev. Rate	Regd. Prev. Rate	No. of Distts. with PR				Distts. under MDT		Cases on Record	Cases under Treat-ment	Cases disch-arged	Cases under MDT
					<2	2-4.9	5	Total	No.	Popul.				
1.	2	3	4	5	6	7	8	9	10	11	12	13	14	15
1.	Andhra Pradesh	663.00	11.3	3.07	10	10	3	23	23	663.00	203521	169662	1190031	99792
2.	Arunachal Pradesh	8.58	3.6	1.52	7	4	Nil	11	Nil	3.10	1305	1198	813	90
3.	Assam	222.94	1.5	0.81	16	2	1	18	1	5.17	18215	18215	13179	6900
4.	Bihar	863.38	5.4	5.22	5	20	14	39	17	429.25	451357	361613	264080	NA
5.	Goa	11.68	5.0	1.05	1	Nil	Nil	1	1	11.68	1228	1228	3917	NA
6.	Gujarat	411.74	2.9	0.54	18	1	Nil	19	19	411.74	22316	21728	128230	20670
7.	Haryana	163.17	.08	0.04	14	Nil	Nil	14	3	46.74	680	680	918	NA
8.	Himachal Pradesh	51.11	1.6	0.77	12	Nil	Nil	12	3	12.94	3956	3956	3299	NA
9.	Jammu & Kashmir	77.18	2.2	1.22	14	Nil	Nil	14	16	30.08	*3720	*3720	*1873	*3582
10.	Karnataka	448.17	6.0	1.60	14	5	1	20	12	346.18	72071	63525	263859	44340
11.	Kerala	290.11	5.3	1.85	10	3	1	14	10	242.70	53932	44045	79209	8671
12.	Madhya Pradesh	661.35	2.3	4.22	18	21	6	45	22	392.70	279286	159948	188864	22865

Contd.

1.	2	3	4	5	6	7	8	9	10	11	12	13	14	15
13.	Maharashtra	737.16	6.2	1.96	18	12	Nil	30	23	621.08	147866	137885	839561	77053
14.	Manipur	18.25	4.5	0.74	8	Nil	Nil	8	3	1.80	1369	1369	4667	531
15.	Meghalaya	17.61	4.6	1.20	3	2	Nil	5	2	6.63	1552	1552	1199	NA
16.	Mizoram	6.86	1.0	0.52	3	Nil	Nil	3	3	6.86	363	363	680	363
17.	Nagaland	12.15	3.9	1.66	5	1	1	7	1	1.28	2026	2026	583	1123
18.	Orissa	315.12	12.1	4.86	2	4	7	13	13	315.12	153267	152041	330106	75212
19.	Punjab	201.90	0.1	0.02	12	Nil	Nil	12	3	53.63	550	549	4651	549
20.	Rajasthan	433.39	1.6	0.45	27	Nil	NIl	27	1	22.87	19911	18324	8026	1861
21.	Sikkim	4.03	7.3	0.27	4	Nil	Nil	4	2	2.75	109	109	348	109
22.	Tamil Nadu	556.38	12.9	3.16	5	12	4	21	21	556.38	176027	163854	1171891	1019801
23.	Tripura	27.44	4.9	0.80	3	Nil	Nil	3	3	27.44	2193	2193	2446	741
24.	Uttar Pradesh	1387.60	3.7	2.56	27	31	5	63	32	749.69	356285	331924	368712	67197
25.	West Bengal	679.82	6.9	3.00	5	10	2	17	15	586.46	203852	119197	529566	73507
26.	Andaman & Nicobar	2.77	4.9	4.60	1	Nil	1	2	1	2.39	1220	1279	1253	57
27.	Chandigarh	6.40	4.7	4.54	Nil	1	Nil	1	1	6.40	2049	2049	13	2049
28.	D & N Haveli	1.38	1.0	2.02	Nil	1	Nil	1	Nil	Nil	280	129	55	129
29.	Daman & Diu	1.01	3.8	2.49	1	1	Nil	2	NA	Nil	252	252	96	52
30.	Delhi	93.70	0.4	0.14	1	Nil	Nil	1	1	93.70	1368	1368	15500	1368
31.	Lakshadweep	0.51	25.0	2.92	Nil	1	Nil	1	1	0.51	151	151	443	151
32.	Pondichery	7.89	15.0	2.48	2	1	1	4	4	7.89	1952	1952	12320	592
	Total	3439.30		2.58	266	143	46	455	257	5685.41	2184299	1787094	5430379	641014

Regd. Prev. Rate = Registered Prevalence Rate
MDT = Multidrug Therapy
NA = Not Available
Popul. = Population
Treat. = Treatment
Distts. = districts
* = Only Jammu Division

APPENDIX 11

GUIDELINES FOR MDT OPERATIONAL PLANNING*

Notations

A subcentre of a control unit covers 20,000 population by a trained leprosy Para-medical worker, similarly a SET Centre covers 25,000 population by a trained leprosy Para-medical worker. The above two types are, on an average, the pattern for a rural area. In the urban area, a trained leprosy urban worker covers about 30,000-70,000 (on an average about 50,000) population, with about 150-350 cases, at the urban leprosy centre. For facilities of operation each two sub-centres, i.e., 40,000-50,000 in a rural area or 60,000 to 140,000 (average 100,000) population in an urban area will form a circuit. Each circuit will have 8-15 clinics or treatment points coverage, daily by the Medical Officer of the control unit, Urban Centre Officer for 20 SET centres or 3-5 urban leprosy centres by a jeep round between 6 am and 1 pm daily. Each Para-medical worker (PMW) will be in charge of 1-2 clinics covering about 4,000-5,000 population. During the previous day on the PMW will contact patients in their homes and motivate them to come to the clinic on the next day at the stipulated place and time. On the clinic day, the PMW will reach the clinic 10 minutes before the clinic time, receive the patients and keep them waiting by talking till the MO comes and gives them treatment. The PMW will check with the case cards or treatment register, the attendance of the patients, and present those to the MO for recording of treatment and checking of clinical and bacteriological findings. After the MO leaves for the next clinic, the PMW with the the treatment record with him, identifies and visits the house of absentee patients and motivates them to come the next day or next month to the clinic as the case may be.

(a) 8-10 circuits will cover 4-5 lakh population. The circuits may

---

* Issued by Government of India for Districtwise Multidrug Treatment Campaign Mobilization of Staff and Schedule of Multidrug Treatment Circuits Pattern.

be termed as A,B,C,D,E,F,G,H,I,J. When a circuit is having daily treatment it may be indicated as A, but when A circuit is given the first pulse treatment, it is marked as A^1 and the second pulse treatment as A^2 and likewise similar notations for other circuits.

(b) There will be 20 PMWs in 20 sub-centres or 20 SET centres and 3-5 PMWs in urban centres. Each of the two workers of two adjoining sub-centres or SET centres of urban centres will from a team for mobilization. They may be termed as team a, b, c, d, e, f, g, h, i, j.

Suppose the actual operation of treatment starts in an area from 1 April, after all preparations in a previous period of 2-3 months of preparatory phase, the schedule of operation and likely mobilization of staff and the timings may be as follows:

Frame:

a	b	c	d	e	f	g	h	i	j	Teams–each of two workers,
1	3	5	7	9	11	13	15	17	19	sub-centres/SET centres, 1
2	4	6	8	10	12	14	16	18	20	PMW each, i.e., total 20 in an unit

A	B	C	D	E	F	G	H	I	J	Circuits–each of 2 sub-centres

1 and 2 form	team a
3 and 4 form	team b
5 and 6 form	team c
and thus up to	team j

Similarly 1 and 2 sub-centres will form 'A' circuit running 8-15 treatment points, 3 and 4 sub-centres will form 'B' circuit and likewise up to 'J' circuit. Total 10 teams and 10 circuits.

Calendar of Activities in Control Unit

Year and Month	Date	No. of days	Routine	Circuit covered	Team mob-ilized	Important works
1st Month	1-2	2	Staff meeting	A	a,c,e,g,i	Shifting of workers and NMS to circuit clinic points on the previous day. Correlation with clinic timings, patients and attendant workers. Motivation of patients by pre-clinic contacts for attending clinic regularly and in time.
	3-16	14	Daily treatment by circuit round 13 13 days multi-bacillary, 14th day both multi and paucibacillary	-do-	-do-	Doctors give treatment to patients kept waiting at each point by PMW and NMS. PMW and NMS follow-up absentee patients after doctors leave for next clinic. Absentee patients are given two days doses on the next day in the clinic or if required by the PMW and NMS by visiting his house, only for a day's treatment at a time and the patient is to attend next day in the clinic. Laboratory and clinical monitoring for toxicity and progress and detection of new

(Contd.)

Year & Month	Date	No. of days	Routine	Circuit covered	Team mobilized	Important works
						cases for treatment. Recording of findings and treatment to be made in Case Cards daily.
	17	1	Follow-up	A	a,c,e,g,i	Absentee patients or those prone to toxicity should be followed up in their houses and given treatment, or hospitalized where necessary.
	18	1	Holiday			
	19-20	2	Pre-clinic contact	B	b,d,f,h,j,	As above
2nd month	21-30 1st month and1-4 of 2nd month	14	Daily treatment as given before	-do-	-do-	-do-
	5	1	Follow-up of absentees	-do-	-do-	-do-
	6-7	2	Holidays			
	8-9	2	Pulse	A^1	a,c,e,g,i	1st day pre-clinic contact by PMW/ NMS. Next day treatment at circuit clinics by MO in jeep rounds. Absentee follow-up and treatment by PMW/NMS after the clinic is over, by home visits.
	10-11	2	Pre-clinic contact	C	a,c,e,g,i	As mentioned earlier for daily treatment

(Contd.)

Year & Month	Date	No. of days	Routine	Circuit covered	Team mob-ilized	Important works
	12-25	14	Daily treatment	-do-	-do-	-do-
	26	1	Follow-up treatment of absentees, etc.	-do-	-do-	-do-
	27-28	2	Holidays			
	29-30	2	Pulse	B^1	b,d,f,h,j	As given before for pulse
3rd Month	31 of 2nd month and 1 of 3rd month	2	-do-	A^2	a,c,e,g,i	-do-
	2-3	2	Pre-clinic contact	D	b,d,f,h,j	As given before for daily treatment
	4-17	14	Daily treatment as given above	-do-	-do-	-do-
	18	1	Follow-up treatment	-do-	-do-	-do-
	19-20	2	Holiday			
	21-22	2	Pulse	C^1	a,c,e,g,i	As mentioned above for pulse
	23-24	2	-do-	B^2	b,d,f,h.j.	-do-
	25-26	2	-do-	A^3	a,c,e,g,i	-do-
	27-28	2	Pre-clinic contact	E	-do-	As given for daily treatment
4th month	28-30 of 3rd Month and 11 of 4th month	14	Daily treatment	-do-	-do-	-do-
	12	1	Absentees treatment	-do-	-do-	-do-
	13-14	2	Pulse	D^1	b,d,f,h,j	As given before for pulse
	15-16	2	Holidays			
	17-18	2	Pulse	C^2	a,c,e,g,i	As given before for pulse

(Contd.)

Year & Month	Date	No. of days	Routine	Circuit covered	Team mobilized	Important works
	19-20	2	Pulse	B^3	b,d,f,h,j	-do-
	21-22	2	Pulse	A^4	a,c,e,g,i	-do-
	23-24	2	Pre-clinic contact	F	b,d,f,h,j	As for daily treatment
5th Month	25-31 of 4th month and 1-7 of 5th month	14	Daily treatment	-do-	-do-	-do-
	8	1	Follow-up absentees	-do-	-do-	-do-
	9-10	2	Pulse	E^1	a,c,e,g,i	As for pulse
	11-12	2	-do-	D^2	b,d,f,h,i	-do-
	13-14	2	Holidays			
	15-16	2	Pulse	C^3	a,c,e,g,i	-do-
	17-18	2	-do-	B^4	b,d,f,h,j	-do-
	19-20	2	-do-	A^5	a,c,e,g,i	-do-
	21-22	2	Pre-clinic contact	G	-do-	As for daily treatment
6th Month	23-31 of 5th month and 1-5 of 6 month	14	Daily treatment	-do-	-do-	-do-
	6	1	Absentees treatment	-do-	-do-	-do-
	7-8	2	Pulse	F^1	b,d,f,h,j	As per pulse.
	9-10	2	-do-	E^2	a,c,e,g,i	-do-
	11-12	2	-do-	D^3	b,d,f,h,j	-do-
	13-14	2	-do-	C^4	a,c,e,g,i	-do-
	15-16	2	-do-	B^5	b,d,f,h,j	As per pulse
	17-18	2	-do-	A^6	a,c,e,g,i	-do-
	19-20	2	Holidays			
	21-22	2	Pre-clinic contact	H	b,d,f,h,j	As for daily treatment

(Contd.)

Year & Month	Date	No. of days	Routine	Circuit covered	Team mobilized	Important works
7th Month	23-30 of 6th month and 1-6 of 7th month	14	Daily treatment	-do-	-do-	-do-
		1	Follow-up of absentees	-do-	-do-	-do-
	8-9	2	Pulse	G^1	a,c,e,g,i	As for pulse
	10-11	2	-do-	F^2	b,d,f,h,j	-do-
	12-13	2	-do-	E^3	a,c,e,g,i	-do-
	14-15	2	-do-	D^4	b,d,f,h,j	-do-
	16-17	2	-do-	C^5	a,c,e,g,i	-do-
	18-19	2	-do-	B^6	b,d,f,h,j	-do-
	20-21	2	-do-	A^7	a,c,e,g,i	-do-
	22-23	2	Holidays			
	24-25	2	Pre-clinic contact	1	-do-	As for daily treatment
8th Month	26-31 of 7th month and 1-8 of 8th month	14	Daily treatment	-do-	-do-	-do-
	9	1	Follow-up of absentees	-do-	-do-	-do-
	10-11	2	Pulse	H^1	b,d,f,h,j	As for pulse
	12-13	2	-do-	G^2	a,c,e,g,i	-do-
	14-15	2	-do-	F^3	b,d,f,h,j	-do-
	16-17	2	-do-	E^1	a,c,e,g,i	As for pulse
	18-19	2	-do-	D^5	b,d,f,h,j	-do-
	20-21	2	-do-	C^6	a,c,e,g,i	-do-
	22-23	2	Follow-up of absentees	B^7	b,d,f,h,j	As pulse treatment
	24-25	2	-do-	A^8	a,c,e,g,i	-do-
	26-27	2	Holidays			
	28-29	2	Pre-clinic contact	J	b,d,f,h,j	As for daily treatment

(Contd.)

Year & Month	Date	No. of days	Routine	Circuit covered	Team mobili-zed	Important works
9th Month	30 of 8th month and 1-13 of 9th month	14	Daily treatment	-do-	-do-	-do-
	14	1	Follow-up absentees treatment	-do-	-do-	-do-
	15-16	2	Pulse	I^1	a,c,e,g,i	As for pulse
	171-8	2	-do-	H^2	b,d,f,h,j	-do-
	19-20	2	-do-	G^3	a,c,e,g,i	-do-
	21-22	2	-do-	F^4	b,d,f,h,j	-do-
	23-24	2	-do-	E^5	a,c,e,g,i	-do-
	25-26	2	-do-	D^6	b,d,f,h,j	-do-
	27-28	2	-do-	C^7	a,c,e,g,i	-do-
	29-30	2	-do-	B^8	b,d,f,h,i	-do-
10th Month	1	1	-do-	A^9	a,c,e,g,i	-do-
	2-4	3	Holidays			
	5-6	2	Pulse	J^1	b,d,f,h,j	-do-
	7-8	2	-do-	I^2	a,c,e,g,i	-do-
	9-10	2	-do-	H^3	b,d,f,h,j	-do-
	11-12	2	-do-	G^1	a,c,e,g,i	As for pulse
	13-14	2	-do-	F^5	b,d,f,h,j	-do-
	15-16	2	-do-	E^6	a,c,e,g,i	-do-
	17-18	2	-do-	D^7	b,d,f,h,i	-do-
	19-20	2	-do-	C^8	a,c,e,g,i	-do-
	21-22	2	-do-	B^9	b,d,f,h,j	-do-
	23-24	2	-do-	A^{10}	a,c,e,g,i	-do-
	25-26	2	Holidays			

This is to be repeated every month till all multibacilary cases have received at least 2 years treatment and paucibacilary cases 6 months treatment covering all active and relapsed cases (Old and New).

As number of paucibacillary cases in a circuit will be large, it is permissible to take all paucibacillary cases in one sub-centre (half circuit) in first 6 months and the remaining paucibacillary cases in second sub-centre in the subsequent 6 months period. Similarly it may be desirable in some circuits to increase the number of drug delivery points when paucibacillary cases are taken up.

APPENDIX 12

RESOLUTION[1]

(On Constitution of National Leprosy Eradication Commission[2])

The Government of India, on 8th July, 1981, vide Resolution No. T.11022/25/81-CCD, constituted a Working Group to formulate an appropriate strategy for undertaking an eradication programme for leprosy in the next 20 years, taking advantage of the present day advances in the chemotherapy of leprosy, the extended reach of mass media, the promise of recent medical research and other relevant factors.

2. In its Report, submitted in March, 1982, the Working Group has recommended an integrated time-bound programme for leprosy eradication, which can help to achieve a synthesis between the preventive, curative and rehabilitative aspects of the problem and its human socio-economic dimensions.

3. The recommendations made by the Working Group have been endorsed by the Joint Conference of the Central Council of Health and Central Family Welfare Council at their meeting held from 18th to 20th August 1982. These have since been considered by the Government and it has been decided that:

I. The existing National Leprosy Control Programme should be redesignated as the National Leprosy Eradication Programme (NLEP)

II. For the guidance and surveillance of the National Leprosy Eradication Programme, a National Leprosy Eradication Commission (NLEC) is set up consisting of the following:

---

1. No. T.11012/3/83-CCD Government of India, Ministry of Health & Family Welfare (Department of Health), New Delhi, the 19th April, 1983.

2. Added for clarification.

Chairman:	Union Minister of Health and Family Welfare
Members:	Union Minister of Finance
	Union Minister of Planning
	Union Minister of Chemicals and Fertilizers
	Union Minister of State for Education and Social Welfare
	Five Chief Ministers of States in Rotation (to be nominated by the Prime Minister)
	Eight eminent Leprologists and Social Workers and others engaged in leprosy control and 'Health for All' Programme in the country. (to be nominated by the Chairman).
Secretary:	Secretary of Ministry of Health and Family Welfare (Ex-officio).

III. (i) As the executive instrument of the National Leprosy Eradication Commission, a National Leprosy Eradication Board (NLEB) is set up consisting of the following:

1.	Secretary for Health and Family Welfare	Chairman
2.	Secretary, Ministry (Department of Expenditure)	Member
3.	Secretary, Ministry of Social Welfare	Member
4.	Secretary, Ministry of Information & Broadcasting	Member
5.	Secretary, Planning Commission	Member
6.	Secretary, Department of Rural Development	Member
7.	Director General of Health Services	Member
8.	Director General, Indian Council of Medical Research	Member
9.	Member for Implementation, Monitoring and Evaluation	Member (whole-time)
10.	Member for Public Participation, Mass Media Mobilisation and Health Education	Member (whole-time)

11.	Member for Research and Development (Deputy Director General concerned in the Indian Council of Medical Research would function as a part-time member for Research and Development)	Member (part-time)
12.	Director of Integrated Programme of Leprosy Eradication	Member Secretary (ex-officio)

III. (ii) In regard to the matters falling within the areas allotted under the Rules of Business to the Ministry of Health and Family Welfare, Ministry of Social Welfare and Ministry of Information and Broadcasting (hereinafter called the relevant Ministries), insofar as the programme activities relating to the prevention, containment and eradication of leprosy and rehabilitation of leprosy patients are concerned, the National Leprosy Eradication Board would have the powers vested in the relevant Ministries in regard to the areas allotted to each of them.

IV. Central Legislation will be initiated to repeal the Lepers Act, 1898 in its application to the Union Territories without legislature. States and Union Territories with Legislatures will also be requested to take similar measure.

V. The National Leprosy Eradication Programme will be implemented as a vertical programme in districts with an endemicity of 5 or above per thousand, until the prevalence rate comes down to below 2.5 per thousand.

VI. Decisions taken by the Government on the other recommendations of the Working Group will be taken up for execution under the guidance of National Leprosy Eradication Commission and through the instrument of National Leprosy Eradication Board. National Leprosy Eradication Board would also further consider, in detail, such of the recommendations which have financial implications. In respect thereof, the National Leprosy Eradication Board will have the power to sanction the schemes, if they are within the financial powers delegated to relevant Ministries. Wherever the schemes are such as exceed the powers delegated to a Ministry/Department of the

Government, the National Leprosy Eradication Board will take the approval of the Expenditure Finance Committee/ Cabinet, as secretary.

VII. Additional resources required during the Sixth Plan period for the implementation of the National Leprosy Eradication Programme have been made available by the Planning Commission.

4. Eradication of Leprosy is part of the national goal of 'Health for All by the year 2000 A.D.'. It is in Government's 20-Point Programme. Government are confident that under the guidance of the National Leprosy Eradication Commission, the National Leprosy Eradication Board will, acting in concert with the State Government/UT Administrations, Voluntary Organisations and all other concerned with this great endeavour, take such initiatives and steps as are necessary to eradicate leprosy by the turn of the country.

S.S. SIDHU
Secretary to the Government of India

APPENDIX 13

RESOLUTION[1]

(On Reconstitution of National Leprosy Eradication Commission[2])

Government of India had set up a National Leprosy Eradication Commission for the guidance and surveillance of National Leprosy Eradication Programme vide Ministry of Health and Family Welfare Resolution No. T.11012/3/83-CCD dated 19th April, 1983. Its term has already expired.

The National Leprosy Eradication Commission is now reconstituted by Government of India with immediate effect. The Composition of the Commission is as under:

Chairman: Union Minister of Health and Family Welfare

Members: (a) **Union Ministers**

1. Union Minister of Finance
2. Union Minister of Planning
3. Union Minister of Industry
4. Minister of State for Welfare

(b) **Chief Ministers of States**

1. Chief Minister of Uttar Pradesh
2. Chief Minister of Madhya Pradesh
3. Chief Minister of Kerala
4. Chief Minister of Maharashtra
5. Chief Minister of Rajasthan

(c) **Eminent Leprologists/Social Workers**

1. Mother Teresa
54-A, Lower Circular Road
Calcutta 700016

---

1. No. T.11016/1/88-CCD; Government of India, Ministry of Health & Family Welfare, New Delhi, the 4th May, 1989.

2. Added for clarification.

2. Dr. B. Sankaran
   Senior Orthopaedic Consultant
   St. Stephen Hospital,
   Tis Hazari,
   Delhi
3. Dr. S.D. Gokhale
   Editor, 'KESARI'
   Pune
4. Dr. R. Ganapati
   Director
   Bombay Leprosy Project
   Purav Marg
   Marathi Vigyan Parishad
   SION-Chuna Batti
   Bombay-22
5. Dr. (Mrs) E.S. Thangaraj
   Leprosy Mission
   Salur-9, Vizianagaram
   Andhra Pradesh
6. Shri S.P. Tare
   Director
   Gandhi Memorial Leprosy Foundation
   Hindi Nagar
   Wardha Maharashtra
7. Dr. E.P. Fritschi
   Schieffelin Leprosy Research and Training Centre
   Karigiri, North Arcot District
   Tamil Nadu
8. Swami Jnanatmananda
   Bharat Sewashram Sangh
   Jamshedpur
   District Singhbhum
   Bihar

Member Secretary: Secretary, Ministry of Health and Family Welfare (ex-officio)

M.S. DAYAL
Additional Secretary (H)
Government of India

APPENDIX 14

PLAN DOCUMENTS: PERTAINING TO LEPROSY

14.1 First Five Year Plan (1951-56)

Leprosy Control Scheme – Scheme for the control of leprosy continued to operate during plan.

14.2 Second Five Year Plan (1956-61)

A Leprosy Advisory Committee was constituted in 1958 to review the working of the Leprosy Control Scheme and to suggest measures for its improvement. By 1958-59, four treatment and study centres and 39 subsidiary centres had been set up.

14.3 Third Five Year Plan (1961-66)

By the end of the second plan, besides facilities for special treatment, 100 centres for leprosy control will have been established. Extensive surveys have been undertaken from these centres and facilities for treatment provided. By 1965-66, it is hoped to increase the number of these centres to over 200. It is also proposed to associate, in anti-leprosy work, a large number of voluntary organisations and social workers; and to bring about greater coordination between various agencies working in this field. It is further envisaged that every hospital and primary health unit in the endemic areas should be organised as a nucleus for leprosy control work.

14.4 Annual Plan (1968-69)

An additional population of 3.7 million was brought under the Programme, bringing the total coverage to 74.1 million by March 1969. The total number of survey, education and treatment (SET) centres rose by 98 to 1130. The number of leprosy control units, however, remained unchanged at 182. Thirty-one voluntary organisations continued to participate in the programme.

14.5 Fourth Five Year Plan (1969-74)

Modern drugs, especially sulphones, can now control leprosy by intensive as well as mass-scale treatment. Emphasis in leprosy control has, therefore, shifted from institutionalisation to case-detection and out-patient treatment with sulphones. During the Third Plan, the programme was reorganised on the basis of experience of the First and Second Plans. Survey, education and treatment (SET) centres were introduced. Each SET centre is attached to a primary health centre, a dispensary or a hospital and covers a population of about 20,000. The basis of approach for the control of leprosy will be to detect cases and treat them. This will prevent the transmission of the disease. By converting the highly infectious cases into non-infectious ones, the quantum of infection will be reduced. It is proposed to establish 100 leprosy control units, 2000 SET centres and 6 training centres for non-medical assistants under the Fourth Plan.

14.6 Fifth Five Year Plan (1974-79)

National Leprosy Control Programme

Leprosy is one of the major public health problems in India. The disease is mostly prevalent in rural areas. It is estimated that about 31 lakhs persons suffer from this disease and is more or less endemic throughout India. It is more prevalent in the Southern and the Eastern States.

372 million of our population are exposed to the risk of contracting leprosy and only 96 million have been covered under the control programme so far. The control programme provides medical care to leprosy patients on domiciliary ambulatory pattern through a network of leprosy control units, survey, examination and treatment centres and training centres for personnel. During the Fourth Plan 57 control units, 342 SET Centres and 39 upgraded subsidiary centres were established against the target of 69 control units, 423 SET Centres and 50 upgraded subsidiary centres respectively. During the Fifth Plan, it is proposed to cover the entire hyper-endemic and moderately-endemic areas (population 276 million) by establishment of 140 control units, 116 upgraded subsidiary centres and 7160 SET Centres.

Leprosy Control

Measures for control of leprosy will be pursued vigorously. Besides financial involvement of State Governments, it would be necessary to encourage voluntary agencies in the implementation of this programme by providing adequate support through grants-in-aid, etc. The functions of leprosy workers would be integrated with other unipurpose workers under the multi-purpose workers scheme but this integration would be carried out last in respect of hyper-endemic leprosy districts. Even thereafter, if necessary, additional workers would be provided to the extent necessary so as to effectively contain this scourge. Adequate financial and other incentives may have to be provided to doctors and other para-professional workers under this programme in view of the social stigma attached to this disease.

14.7 Sixth Five Year Plan (1980-85)

The leprosy control programme will be intensified in the Plan towards the objective of its eradication as early as possible. The programme will be directed towards the following objectives:

(a) To cover the entire endemic population of the country to the extent of 90 per cent by 1985 and 100 per cent by 1990 with a corresponding step up in disease arrested cases from present level of 20 per cent to 40 per cent in 1985 and 60 per cent in 1990.

(b) To introduce newer drugs, multi-drug therapy and specially supervised treatment of infectious cases and epidemiological surveillance by a network of early detection measures.

(c) To provide medico-surgical facilities to leprosy patients for rehabilitation through reconstructive surgery, physiotherapy, occupational therapy, jobs and tools adoption, etc.

(d) To improve and extend training facilities in leprosy through training centres, Regional Leprosy Training-cum-Referral Institutes and workshops.

(e) Encourage the participation of voluntary agencies through financial support. Public education and mass publicity will be stepped up to remove the social stigma attached to the disease.

14.8 Seventh Five Year Plan (1985-90)

The National Leprosy Control Programme has been further augmented and converted into a National Leprosy Eradication Programme, based on the strategies and policies formulated by a high level committee. 350 million people living in areas of the country where the disease is endemic have been covered under the programme. A total of 3 million cases are under active treatment against an estimated 4 million leprosy affected patients. The Sixth Plan target of 90 per cent case detection could not thus be fully achieved.

14.9 Eighth Five Year Plan (1992-97)

Programmes for Control of Communicable Diseases

A number of national programmes for eradication/control of communicable diseases have been initiated in the country since the early years of planning. Most of the control/eradication programmes for communicable diseases have been in operation since last several plans at huge financial cost. With a few exceptions, however, no national level comprehensive review/evaluation of these programmes have been undertaken. During the Eighth Plan the following strategies will be followed for control of communicable diseases:

(i) National level review of the ongoing control/eradication programe to assess the current strategies and their impact on the disease status.
(ii) Ensuring sufficient supplies and logistic support including mobility for carrying out the programmes.
(iii) Establishment of epidemiological-cum-surveillance centres at district/regional levels and improvement of health management information system for continuous monitoring of the disease situation and taking appropriate and prompt action.
(iv) Intersectoral coordination will be strengthened with departments of public health engineering, local bodies, like municipalities, Ministries of Information and Broadcasting, Women and Child Welfare, Water Resources, etc., for control of vector borne and other diseases.

(v) The Information, Education and and Communication (IEC) activities within each programme would be given special attention for enlisting community participation, which constitutes one of the weakest links, for carrying out the disease control programmes.

(vi) Strategy of training of staff at horizontal level, both within the primary health care and higher level, is essential.

(vii) Training in epidemiology is woefully inadequate in the country. Unless this situation is rectified decisions regarding control of communicable diseases and its implementation will be handled by the group of professionals and para-professionals who are not sufficiently equipped to do so with its attendant consequences. Specialised institutions/departments to carry out both pre-service and in-service training in epidemiology for different category of staff will be created and the existing ones strengthened.

Leprosy Eradication

The approach, under this 100 per cent Centrally Sponsored Scheme has been early case detection and domiciliary treatment and health education. Multi Drugs Therapy (MDT) has been introduced in all 201 endemic districts and 41 low endemic districts (till March 1991) for case treatment. The programme has shown steady progress in achieving its objectives during the Seventh Plan.

Within the Leprosy Eradication Programme the following activities will be pursued:

(i) Creation of additional physical facilities in all the endemic districts.

(ii) Extension of MDT to remaining endemic districts and in low endemic districts in phases.

(iii) Training of the PHC staff in leprosy eradication activities, both in endemic and low endemic districts, with the aim of preparing them to take over the responsibility of leprosy eradication activities following reduction in the prevalence and incidence of the disease.

(iv) Creation of vocational and rehabilitation facilities for the patients declared cured in those districts which have been under MDT for more than 5 years.

APPENDIX 15

NATIONAL PROFILE OF LEPROSY

With the population of 843.9 million as determined by the 1991 Census, India is estimated to have 2.8 to 3.0 million patients suffering from leprosy, accounting for nearly one-third of the global disease load.

There has been a progressive decrease in the number of cases as more and more districts came under the MDT umbrella. Currently, 201 of the 455 districts in the country are under the MDT cover, providing protection to nearly 470.4 million people of these 66 districts are under the modified MDT programme. The new cases detected during April 1991 were 2.0 million against 3.38 million found in 1987. About 6.0 million patients had been discharged by the end of March, 1991 since the programme began.

Since 1988, the number of leprosy patients cured each year have exceeded those detected, thus moving towards the target of arresting the disease by the year 2000 A.D. The projected yearly targets for case detection and cure as also the cases at the end of each year up to the year 2000 are presented in Table A15.1.

TABLE A15.1: Projected yearly targets for case-detection and cure

(Numbers in thousand)

Year	No. of cases at the beginning of the year	New cases	No. of Discharges		No. of cases at at the end of the year
			MDT	Monotherapy death, other reasons	
1991	2120	+450	−500	−300	1770
1992	1770	+420	−650	−250	1290
1993	1290	+400	−500	−200	990
1994	990	+370	−500	−100	760
1995	760	+320	−500	−50	530
1996	530	+280	−450	−30	330
1997	330	+240	−380	−20	170
1998	170	+220	−250	−20	120
1999	120	+150	−200	−10	60
2000	60	+120	−150	−10	20

ABBREVIATED VOLUNTARY MUSCLE TESTING[1]

These tests are carried out on the muscles of the face, hands, and legs. The scoring is graded from 0-5 (Table A16.1).

TABLE A16.1: Definitions of muscle power test (VMT) scoring grades

Grade	Eyelids	Hand muscles*	Dorsiflexion of foot*
5	Normal power	normal range of movement, normal power	normal power
4	weak but eyelids close	normal range of movement, less than normal power	active movement against gravity and resistance
3	slight lag-ophthalmos	normal range of movement against slight or no resistance	active movement against gravity
2	marked lag-ophthalmos	reduced range of movement when there is no resistance	active movement with gravity eliminated
1	flicker of movement	muscle flicker, no (or minimal) joint movement	flicker or trace of contraction
0	complete paralysis	complete paralysis	no contraction

* If there is restriction of passive movement, "normal range" is taken to be the range of passive movement.

(1) *Facial nerve – orbicular muscle of the eye.*

(a) *Blink test*. When the patient blinks spontaneously it is observed whether or not the upper lid touches the lower lid. The finding is recorded.

---

1. *Source*: WHO, 1988, *A Guide to Leprosy Control*, 2nd ed, World Health Organization, Geneva.

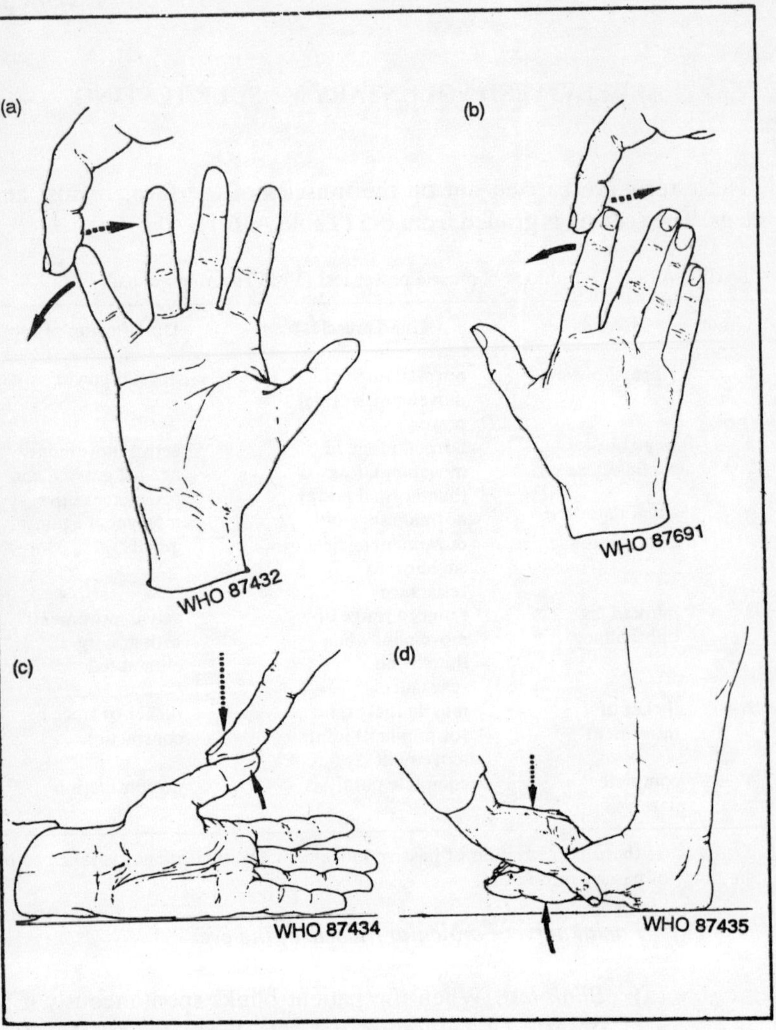

FIG. A16.1: Method of testing for muscle power (VMT)

(a) Abductor muscle of the little finger (ulnar nerve)
(b) First dorsal interosseous muscle (ulnar nerve)
(c) Short abductor muscle of the thumb (median nerve)
(d) Anterior tibial muscle (lateral popliteal nerve)

(b) *Voluntary muscle test*. The patient is asked to shut the eyes as tightly as possible. The muscle strength is recorded.

(2) *Ulnar nerve – abductor muscle of the little finger* [Fig. A16.1 (a)]. The back of the hand and fingers are placed flat on a table. The patient abducts the little finger against resistance. The muscle strength is recorded.
(3) *Ulnar nerve – first dorsal interosseous muscle* [Fig. A16.1 (b)]. The palm of the hand and the fingers are placed flat on a table. The patient abducts the index finger against resistance. The muscle strength is recorded.
(4) *Median nerve – short abductor muscle of the thumb* [Fig. A16.1 (c)]. The back of the hand and fingers are placed flat on a table. The patient abducts the thumb vertically upwards, at right angles to the palm of the hand, against resistance. The muscle strength is recorded.
(5) *Lateral popliteal nerve – anterior tibial muscle* [Fig. A16.1 (d)]. The patient dorsiflexes the foot against resistance. The muscle power is recorded.

CLASSIFICATION OF DISABILITIES*

The WHO Expert Committee on Leprosy, in its fifth report (WHO, 1970) commented that the disability grading system formulated in 1970 (WHO, 1977) was "rather beyond the comprehension of primary health workers". It is evident that no one system of grading will meet all requirements. A simple three-grade (0, 1 and 2) system of classification is suggested below, primarily for collection of general data regarding disabilities and impairments.

Hands and Feet

Grade 0 : no anaesthesia, no visible deformity or damage.
Grade 1 : anaesthesia present, but no visible deformity or damage.
Grade 2 : visible deformity or damage present.

Each hand and foot should be assessed and graded separately. "Damage" in this context includes ulceration, shortening, disorganization, stiffness, and loss of part or all of the hand or foot.

It may be noted that the proposed grades 0 and 1 are the same as the previous grades 0 and 1 respectively; the proposed grade 2 includes the previous grades 2 and 3.

If any disability found in the patient is due to causes other than leprosy, this fact should be noted.

Eyes

The following three-grade classification (grades 0-2) is recommended:

---

* *Source:* WHO, 1988, *A Guide to Leprosy Control*, 2nd ed., World Health Organization, Geneva.

Grade 0 : no eye problems due to leprosy; no evidence of visual loss.

Grade 1 : eye problems due to leprosy present, but vision not severely affected as a result (vision 6/60 or better; can count fingers at six metres).

Grade 2 : severe visual impairment (vision worse than 6/60; inability to count fingers at six metres).

Eye problems due to leprosy include corneal anaesthesia, lagophthalmos, and iridocyclitis.

Each eye should be assessed and classified separately.

If any disability found in the patient is due to any cause other than leprosy, this fact should be noted.

Overall grading of the patient

It will often be necessary to provide information on an overall disability grading for the patient. In that case, the highest value of the leprosy disability grade for any part should be taken as the overall disability grading of the patient.

REFERENCES

1. WHO, 1970, Technical Report Series No. 459.
2. WHO, 1977, Technical Report Series No. 607.

REPORT OF WORKSHOP ON TRAINING OF UNDERGRADUATE MEDICAL STUDENTS IN LEPROSY, 1979

A Workshop sponsored jointly by the Medical Council of India and the Gandhi Memorial Leprosy Foundation, was held to draw up a detailed programme of curriculum and training requirements in leprosy for the undergraduate medical students, at the All India Institute of Hygiene and Public Health, Calcutta on February 23-24, 1979.

The Workshop began at 11.00 A.M. on 23rd February when following were present:

1. Dr. B. Mukhopadhaya
   Vice-President
   Medical Council of India
   Saidpur Road
   Patna (*Chairman*)
2. Dr. D.B. Bisht
   Dy. Director-General of Health Services
   New Delhi
3. Dr. M.D. Gupte
   Acting Director
   Gandhi Memorial Leprosy Foundation
   Wardha
4. Dr. N.S. Deodhar
   Director
   All India Institute of Hygiene and Public Health
   Calcutta
5. Dr. P.V. Sathe
   Professor of Dermatology
   Govt. Medical College
   Aurangabad

6. Dr. B.M.S. Bedi
   Professor of Dermatology
   Govt. Medical College
   Panaji (Goa)
7. Dr. P. Kapoor
   Joint Director of Health Services (Leprosy)
   Poona
8. Dr. R.N. Srivastava
   Professor & Head of the Department of Social & Preventive Medicine
   M.L.B. Medical College
   Jhansi
9. Dr. U.B. Krishnan
   Secretary
   Medical Council of India
   New Delhi (*Convener*)

Following two participants had conveyed their inability to attend on 23rd due to cancellation of Madras-Calcutta Flight. They joined the Workshop on 24th February:

10. Dr. A.S. Thambiah
    Professor of Dermatology
    Madras Medical College
    Madras
11. Dr. J.M. Boopalraj
    Assistant Professor
    Deptt. of Leprosy
    Medical College, Madras

The participants discussed all aspects of training of medical undergraduates, involvement of teachers of Medical Colleges in teaching of leprosy, refresher courses for general medical practitioners and other related matters and decided as follows:

I. Syllabus

It was generally recognised that there were lacunae in the teaching of leprosy in undergraduate curriculum and there was scope for strengthening the training programme.

FOR UNDERGRADUATE MEDICAL STUDENTS

Objectives:

The participants felt that the undergraduate medical students at the end of 4½ years course:

(i) should know the natural history and clinical manifestations so as to suspect and diagnose leprosy in all stages especially in the early stage;
(ii) should be able to manage therapy of the disease and its complications comprehensively;
(iii) be conversant with social pathology of the disease and have compassionate but scientific attitude towards leprosy patients; and
(iv) should know the principles of prevention and control of leprosy.

Suggested syllabus for training

(a) *Clinical Aspects*: Clinical spectrum, diagnosis in all stages particularly in early stage; classification; demonstration of slit and scrape method; laboratory diagnosis; differential diagnosis, natural course; complications; care of feet, hands, etc., by patient; treatment with drugs; type of reactions and their management; lepromin test; social aspects of leprosy.

(b) *Pathological and Microbiological Aspects*: Gross histopathology of leprosy, morphology and characteristics of *M. Leprae,* demonstration of effects on various tissues and organs.

(c) *Pharmacological Aspects*: Anti-leprosy drugs.

(d) *Surgical Aspects*: Aetiology and early detection of injuries and ulcers; management of ulcers; common deformities, their prevention and management including surgical correction; ophthalmic complications and their management; demonstration of physiotherapy in leprosy.

(e) *Preventive and Social Medicine Aspects*: Epidemiology of leprosy; problems in case detection and case holding; prevention and control; immunoprophylaxis and chemoprophylaxis; social factors in leprosy; health education of the patient, relatives and society in general; rehabilitation, National Leprosy Control Programme Organisation, role to be played by general medical practitioner and medical officer at primary health centre, field demonstration of leprosy control programme; visit to the home of a leprosy patient to study the patient and his family.

It was recommended that the existing department of dermatology should be coordinating department for implementing this programme on items (a) to (e).

(f) At the end of post-examination internship period a medical student:

(i) should know how to work with commonly available facilities at Primary Health Centres for prevention and total management of leprosy.
(ii) should know role of a doctor in NLCP, and
(iii) should acquire skills and know application of health education techniques at individual, family and community level for prevention and control of leprosy.

Out of the period of six months' rural internship, the medical student should have participating experience in leprosy control programme for a period of 15 days.

The Medical Council of India was requested to circulate these recommendations as recommendations of the Medical Council of India to all the Medical Colleges in India.

II. Involvement of Teachers of Medical Colleges in Teaching of Leprosy

It was recommended that teachers from different disciplines of medical colleges be approached through various modalities to know their views and to stimulate them to make the teaching programme in leprosy more effective and implement the suggested programme. One such modality could be to bring together medical teachers from concerned disciplines of two or three medical colleges for one day symposium. Such a programme will be organised by a senior person with experience in leprosy work. Another modality would be to have a seminar discussion by a local active teacher supplemented and supported by a senior person from outside the institute.

It is recommended that Gandhi Memorial Leprosy Foundation be requested to devise, implement and evaluate such programmes by itself or in collaboration with Central or State Government, Medical Council of India, universities, other voluntary agencies, etc. After gaining experience of the effectiveness of different modalities and taking into consideration local conditions, suitable programmes could be developed.

III. Continuing Education

(a) The Workshop also reviewed the question of organising and conducting refresher/orientation courses for the general medical practitioners to bring them up to date on the modern concepts for the diagnosis and treatment of leprosy. The Workshop took note of the efforts made in this regard by the Gandhi Memorial Leprosy Foundation.

(b) *Orientation Training in Leprosy for Medical Officers of Primary Health Centres*: Experience of the six day programme of the Gandhi Memorial Leprosy Foundation in training medical officers of Primary Health Centres in Wardha District was presented by Dr. M.D. Gupte. Dr. Gupte was requested to send a detailed scheme on this subject to Dr. Bisht, Dy. Director General, Health Services.

The Workshop then ended with a vote of thanks to the Chair.

APPENDIX 19

EXTRACTS FROM DRAFT PAPER ON REVISED CURRICULUM FOR UNDERGRADUATE MEDICAL EDUCATION, 1992*

CURRICULUM: CLINICAL SUBJECTS

Dermatology and Venereology

Goal

The aim of teaching the undergraduate student in Dermatology, Venereology and Leprology is to impart such knowledge and skills that may enable him to diagnose and treat common ailments, and to refer rare diseases, or complications/unusual manifestations of common diseases, to the specialist.

Objectives

Knowledge

At the end of the course of Dermato-venereology and Leprology, the student should be able to:

1. demonstrate sound knowledge of common diseases, their clinical manifestations, including emergent situations and of investigative procedures to confirm their diagnosis;
2. demonstrate comprehensive knowledge of various modes of topical therapy;
3. describe the mode of action of commonly used drugs, their doses, side-effects/toxicity, indications and contra-indications and interactions;

---

* Source: Report of the Committee under the Chairmanship of Prof. S.K. Kacker, appointed by the Medical Council of India, New Delhi.

4. describe commonly used modes of management including the medicinal and surgical procedures available for the treatment of various diseases, and to offer a comprehensive plan of management for a given disorder;

Skills

The student should be able to:

1. interview the patient, elicit relevant and correct information, and describe the history in a chronological order;
2. conduct clinical examination, elicit and interpret physical findings, and diagnose common disorders and emergencies;
3. perform simple, routine investigative and office procedures required for making the bed-side diagnosis, especially the examination of scrapings for fungus, preparation of slit smears and staining for AFB for leprosy patients, and for STD cases;
4. take a skin biopsy for diagnostic purposes;
5. manage common diseases recognizing the need for referral for specialized care, in case of inappropriateness of therapeutic response.

Alleinative Track for Professional Career

CLINICAL TRAINING SCHEDULE

Clinical training programme for the two years six months period will be as follows:

Field Practice Area:
Orientation to community medicine, National health programmes and health activities directed for goal of health for all by 2000. (36 weeks).
Maternal and Child Health Programmes
including posting in Maternity ward, pediatrics (24 weeks)

Family Medicine.

medicine	:	12-16 weeks	
surgery	:	12-16 weeks	
emergency	:	4-6 weeks	(60 weeks)

Framing of this training programme will inculcate technical, scientific and management abilities in students so as to enable them to work effectively in comprehensive health system based on primary health care in the country.

Act as Primary Care Physician/Surgeon/Obst Gyn

I Diagnose correctly and give appropriate treatment for

Sorethroat, Upper respiratory infections
Pneumonia, Asthama
P.u.o. malaria, Kalazar, Filiaria
Typhoid, Tuberculosis, Amoebiasis
Rheumatic fever, Arthritis
Meningitis
Convulsions, Coma
Urinary tract infection, Anuria
Visceral colic
Diarrhoea, Dehydration
Nutritional deficiencies
Worm infections

peptic ulcer and its complications
Jaundice, hepatitis

Anaemia, Bleeding disorders
Hypertension, Heart failure
Diabetes Mellitus

Snake bite
Heart stroke
Electric Shock
Drowning

Ulcer, Abcesse
Trauma
Head injuries
Acute Abdomen
Internal and External Haemorhage, Shock
Burns
Simple fractures, Dislocations

Dermatology

Allergic states
Scabies

Fungal infections
Leprosy
Psychiatry

Acute Psychiatric illness, Hysteria, Mania,
Anxiety, Depression
Common poisonings

ENT/EYE

Sinusitis
Otitis media
Epistaxis
Eye infections, Trauma, Foreign body.

DISCIPLINE ORIENTED INTERNSHIP

Community Medicine

Interns should acquire skills to deal effectively with an individual and the community in the context of primary health care. This is to be achieved by hands on experience in the district hospital and primary health centre.

I **Community Health Centre/District Hospital/Attachment to G.P.**

(1) During this period of internship, acquire
  a. clinical competence for diagnosis of common ailments, use of bed side investigation and primary care techniques
  b. gain information on 'Essential drugs' and their usage
  c. Recognise medical emergencies, resuscitate institute initial treatment and refer to suitable institution.

(2) Undergo specific Governmeint of India/Ministry of Health and Family Welfare approved training using prescribed training manual for Medical Officers in all National Health Programmes (e.g., child survival and safe motherhood — EPI, CDD, ARI, FP Microntrate, ANC, safe delivery, TB, Leprosy and others as recommended by Ministry of Health and Family Welfare).

a. Gain full expertise in immunisation against infectious disease.
b. participate in programmes in prevention and control of locally prevalent (endemic diseases including nutritional disorders)
c. Learn skills first hand in family planning procedures.
d. Learn the management of National Health Programmes.

(3) Be capable of conducting a survey, and employ its finding as a measure towards arriving at a community diagnosis.

(4) a. conduct programmes on health education
b. gain capabilities to use AV aids
c. acquire capability of utilization of scientific information for promotion of community health.

(5) Be capable of establishing linkages with other agencies as water supply, food distribution and other environmental/social agencies.
(6) Acquire quality of being professional with dedication, resourcefulness and leadership.
(7) To acquire managerial skill, relegation of duties to paramedical staff, and other health professionals.

APPENDIX 20

BACKGROUND PAPER OF WORKSHOP OF NEED BASED CURRICULUM

for Undergraduate Medical Education, Medical Council of India, August 28-29, 1992

Medical Council of India constituted a committee for review of curriculum and for introducing some innovations for the undergraduate medical courses. This committee was to address itself to recommend a curriculum:

(a) That is need based for the country.
(b) That provides a balance between new information on medical sciences and the social applications for medicine, *i.e.*, present day HiTech diagnostic, therapeutic applications should not overide the the humanistic aspects of the profession.
(c) That provides competency in skills than mere theoretical knowledge.
(d) That will provide a first hand experience in clinical care and sharing of responsibilities, preferably at a setting away from the teaching hospitals during the internship training.

To evolve a strategy for implementation of above objectives, proposal of a structured examination at national level to ensure that the curriculum contents are covered, was to be framed.

WHO directions for orientation in medical education state:[1]

(a) Need to view medical education as well as the health care system as a part of social development.
(b) Need to coordinate medical education with the health care system.
(c) Need to correct the over-emphasis on only disease oriented and curative aspects of medicine and to have a more holistic ap-

---

1. SEARO-Regional Publication No. 18, 1988.

proach covering promotive, preventive, curative and rehabilitative aspects.

(d) Need to correct the imbalance between the tertiary care hospital-based medical education to a community-based one.

(e) Need to correct the over emphasis on the use of teacher-oriented to learner-oriented methods which would include self-initiated, self-directed learning and self-evaluation.

(f) Need to correct a narrowly discipline oriented teaching to include a problem-oriented approach.

(g) Need to shift the emphasis from theoretically oriented teaching to experiential learning.

A committee of 20 members was constituted for this purpose in October 1991. The committee appointed a working group to draft recommendations for the evolution of a revised curriculum. The working group has met on 5 occasions, incorporated views of International agencies, e.g., WHO, UNICEF, National agencies, as Ministry of Health, ICMR, NIHFW, and many other eminent specialists in the field of medical education.

A draft so prepared has been circulated to all members of the committee.

During discussions at different stages, main issues raised have been categoried as Contents, Time Allocation, Methodology, Evaluation, Internship. A questionnaire has been formulated as to elicit consensus on the different possibilities defining scope of each of the above items. Again, in order to prepare the medical graduate for general practice or as functionary to provide care in the community, an Alternative Track after pre-clinical, paraclinical training has been designed. The focus of the training in these courses will be on general practice in community setting, with capabilities of providing primary and secondary care. There will be a significant component for training in Mother and Child Health Care and family welfare programmes. Inputs will be provided to work with a health care team to achieve fulfillment of national health programmes and to participate in health education activities in the community.

The opportunities for those who elect this track will be equivalent to those who continue as physicians to be specialists or to take postgraduate courses.

Medical graduation degree in both cases will be MBBS. While physicians/specialist will opt for speciality training (post-graduation in medicine, surgery, obstetrics/gynaecology, pediatrics, orthopaedics, Ophthalmolgy, etc.) those in alternative track can take postgraduation in Family Medicine, MCH or community medicine. This would meet the central theme of 'Health for all by 2000 A.D.' of WHO, "to open the scope for universal coverage with primary care that is relevant, effective acceptable and affordable in terms of the need, culture, interests and resources of each community."

Given the political will and support from the State Governments, primary care physicians can contribute much more towards national health status and national programmes.

There will be option on part of the medical college to adopt this alternative educational training programme, with given adequate infrastructure and terms of references indicated. Recognition criteria of Medical Council of India (MCI) will be modified for such colleges.

The meeting invites your candid views on the subject, provides you a forum for open discussion and to guide the committee for arriving at a consensus so that a future training programme for the under graduates is made more relevant to national needs, more practical in learning skills and be objectively evaluable at a national level. It should also promote incentives so that those aspiring for higher academic and professional training can pursue this and improve future professional career.

It should be recognised that the recommendations of MCI are guidelines or a framework in which each college can evolve a curriculum in accordance with their faculty, and outreach area of health care and resources.

It is desirable that centres of medical education create modules for health care and work in liaison with other state health agencies for a concerted effort to improve the health status of the nation.

CONCLUSIONS AND RECOMMENDATIONS OF WHO – GOVERNMENT OF INDIA FOURTH INDEPENDENT EVALUATION, 1991

1. Commendable as the new case detection, MDT coverage and release of treated cases were, these activities needed to be strengthened in general and particularly, in States whose performance was not so good in this regard. Case detection should be activated through mass surveys, school surveys and house to house searches. Frontline workers should be encouraged to make greater efforts for retrieval of drug defaulters.
2. Detailed epidemiological studies should be initiated in districts completing 5 years of MDT implementation, where the prevalence rate markedly declined and yet the proportion of child cases among the new cases showed an increase and there was no appreciable decline in the new case detection rates.
3. Monitoring of multi-drug therapy be augmented to detect drug resistance and post RFT surveillance strengthened.
4. Untrained staff in sufficient numbers existed within the programme at all levels. Time bound, phased leprosy training should be arranged for all categories of untrained staff. DLOs and MOs must be trained both in the management of the programme and the clinical aspects of leprosy to improve guidance and supervision of the field workers.
5. The training centres were grossly underutilized. The training capacity should be fully consumed and extended to look after the needs of neighbouring States without such centers.
6. An extensive data was collected through the net-work of information reporting system. Not much use was made of it for improving the programme performance. Basic workshops for all health workers in data collection, compilation, analysis and usage should be organised to remove this weakness. The supervisory and paramedical staff be given orientation training in programme awareness creation amongst the public.

7. The programme suffered from significant number of vacancies at each level. These should be filled at the earliest possible. Particular attention need be paid to the posts of physiotherapist, laboratory technicians and health educators. States, like West Bengal may be requested to create the posts of health educators and physiotherapists that were almost non-existent.
8. Bacteriological surveillance continued to be a weak link in the programme. The laboratory services must be improved by:

   (a) immediately filling up the existing vacancies;
   (b) expeditious training of the untrained laboratory technicians by organizing crash courses in skin smear preparation and reading;
   (c) provision of good workable microscopes; and
   (d) creation of new posts of smear technicians in keeping with the work load.

   It is for consideration if the work load of existing laboratory technicians be reduced by limiting the skin smear examination only to the multibacillary cases.

9. Regular and adequate supply of anti-leprosy drugs is a prerequisite for implementation of MDT. Drug shortage, particularly of clofazimine and rifampicin, affected several of the districts and units. Buffer stocks of these drugs at the State headquarters to last at least for 3 months should be ensured. Drug requirements at all State and lower levels should be preplanned and periodically reviewed.
10. The State Leprosy Officers should be at least of the rank of a State joint director, must be exposed to leprosy work, and must exercise administrative and financial independence. Frequent transfers of the State Leprosy Officer, the District Leprosy Officer and Medical Officers should be avoided, particularly of those who were trained and possessed experience in leprosy.
11. The replacement of condemned vehicles should be an automatic and expeditious process. Mobility of all the staff should be assured by providing vehicles and adequate funds for POL. Imposing governmental restriction on touring adversely affected supervision. States, doing so, may be requested to waive such restrictions.

12. Working of temporary hospitalization units must be radically activated. Their possession of full complement of trained staff must be assured to promote disability prevention by bringing them under the administrative control of the SLO/DLO, as also their utilization for the purpose they were created for.
13. The SSAUs should be looked into both in respect to their staffing and workload. With rapidly advancing MDT coverage in the country, true disease prevalence should be worked out for States that were attended to decades ago. So called low endemic areas should be focused on in a phased manner.
14. Under the impact of MDT as a dramatic decline occurred in case load, continued emphasis to the endemic districts left the non-endemic ones in relative neglect. Extension of MDT to these area should be expeditiously considered.
15. Integration of leprosy services with primary health care presented certain difficulties as seen in Rajasthan and Himachal Pradesh, while the extension of modified multidrug treatment scheme was beset with other local problems. These should be carefully considered before pushing forward these schemes.
16. Growing awareness of the programme in the community and the sharp rise in the rate of voluntary reporting were encouraging. Efforts at health education, however, should be further augmented particularly, with greater emphasis on imparting knowledge of leprosy to the people.

IDENTIFICATION OF TASKS AT DIFFERENT PHC LEVELS*

Level of PHC System	*Tasks*
Home level	Awareness and recognition of skin symptoms, suspicion of leprosy. Social acceptance of leprosy and encouragement and support of the patient at home. Motivation for continuation of treatment
Community level (community health worker, at home, in the community and in collaboration with first level health facility)	Suspicion of symptoms and signs of leprosy Referral of persons with lesions suspicious of leprosy to health facility Monitor treatment Provide social and moral support to patients and family members and assist in rehabilitation of patients Suspect leprosy reactions, side-effects of drugs and referral health education - early sings - treatment - follow-up - advice on complications (self-care) - motivation/moral support

(Contd.)

---

* WHO/CDS/LEP/863

Level of PHC System	*Tasks*
	Simple data collection and reporting (e.g., when patients move out of the village or die) Drug delivery (in special cases)
First level health facility (health centre or equivalent)	Diagnosis of leprosy and classification (MB or PB) based on clinical and bacteriolo-gical examination (smear-taking should be done at this level. The examination of smears may take place at the first referral level) Initiation and supervision of treatment Diagnosis of complications and their treatment (ulcers) or referral (severe reactions) Training and supervision of community health workers. Education and information of the patients and families regarding treatment/follow-up and prevention of disabilities Recording and reporting Surveillance of patients after release from chemotherapy.
First referral level (district hospital/ district) health administration	Smear examination Treatment of severe complications including hospital admission Training and supervision of first level health facility Planning and organizing district level leprosy control activities Monitoring and evaluation of first level health facility Quality Control of performance of first level health facilities. Recording and Reporting

(Contd.)

Level of PHC System	*Tasks*
Higher levels (e.g. provincial, regional, zonal, national)	Specialization regarding management of problem cases Policy decision Priority setting Targets establishment Resource estimation and allocation Overall planning of national programme Preparation of standards and guidelines Training of regional/provincial level managers Supervision and coordination Management of logistic support Epidemiological surveillance Operational research Monitoring and evaluation

APPENDIX 23

RESOLUTION OF FORTY-FOURTH WORLD HEALTH ASSEMBLY[1]

Leprosy

The Forty-fourth World Health Assembly,

Having considered the report of the Director-General on leprosy;

Recalling resolution WHA40.35 and previous resolutions of the Health Assembly and the Executive Board on leprosy;

Noting with satisfaction the significant progress made during the past five years with multidrug therapy for leprosy control and with case-finding in the majority of Member States where leprosy is endemic — progress which has led to reductions in disease prevalence;

Recognizing the substantial and increasing support for leprosy control being provided by nongovernmental and other donor organizations;

Aware of the increasingly high priority accorded by several Member States to the elimination of leprosy as a public health problem;

Further aware of the opportunities to reduce disabilities due to leprosy through early case-detection, multidrug therapy and increased emphasis on managerial capabilities within leprosy control programmes and on disability prevention;

1. DECLARES WHO's commitment to continuing to promote the use of all control measures including multidrug therapy together with case-finding in order to attain the global elimination[2] of leprosy as a public health problem by the year 2000;
2. URGES Member States in which leprosy is endemic:
   (1) to further increase or maintain their political commitment and give high priority to leprosy control so that the global elimination of leprosy as a public health problem is achieved by the year 2000;

---

1. Agenda Item 17.2, WHA 44.A, May 13, 1991.

2. Elimination of leprosy as a public health problem is defined as the reduction of prevalence to a level below one case per 10,000 population.

(2) to strengthen managerial capabilities within leprosy programmes, particularly at the intermediate level, and to improve training in leprosy for health workers at all levels, including medical students and student nurses;
(3) to ensure that coverage of multidrug therapy is maintained at the highest level possible and that patients comply with treatment;
(4) to strengthen case-finding activities through various approaches, including health education, community participation and training of health workers;
(5) to integrate leprosy control within general health services and provide appropriate social and economic rehabilitation measures as soon as possible in accordance with local realities;
(6) to improve national information systems in order to facilitate monitoring and evaluation of the elimination of leprosy;
(7) to coordinate the technical and financial resources made available for leprosy control by international and nongovernmental organizations so that they are utilized in the best way;

3. REQUESTS the Director-General:
(1) to strengthen technical support to Member States for the implementation of multidrug therapy together with case-finding so as to achieve the global elimination of leprosy as a public health problem by the year 2000;
(2) to continue to mobilize and coordinate scientific, technical and additional financial resources for implementing multidrug therapy together with case-finding, disability prevention and social and economic rehabilitation;
(3) to continue to strengthen national capabilities for leprosy control through support for training activities;
(4) to continue to support research for the development of improved drugs, diagnostic tools and vaccines through the Special Programme for Research and Training in Tropical Diseases;
(5) to promote further coordination with Member States and nongovernmental organizations in order to achieve the global elimination of leprosy as a public health problem by the year 2000;
(6) to keep the Executive Board and the Health Assembly informed of the progress made.

(Eleventh plenary meeting, 13 May 1991 A44/VR/11)

APPENDIX 24

VOLUNTARY ORGANISATIONS AND THEIR ACTIVITIES IN THE FIELD OF LEPROSY ERADICATION IN INDIA*

TABLE A24.1: Voluntary Organisations: Year of Commencement and Annual Budget

Sl. No.	Name of voluntary organisation	Year of commen-cement	Annual budget (Rs. in lakhs)
1.	2	3	4
	ANDHRA PRADESH		
1.	Assissi Sisters of Assissi Nagar, Konkepudi, Via Pedana, Distt. Krishna	1981	0.45
2.	Comprehensive Health Care Unit, Parvatipuram, Dist. Krishna	1973	3.00
3.	Hind Kusht Nivaran Sangh, Huzurabad, Jammigunta, Dist. Krimnagar-505122	1968	7.41
4.	Health Centre, Asha Niketan, Vengal Rao Nagar, Kavali, Nellore Distt.	1971	3.10
5.	Greater Tenali Leprosy Treatment and Health Education Scheme, Gandhinagar Tenali, Dist. Guntur	1982	4.12
6.	*St. Joseph Leprosy Rehabilitation Centre, PO Timmarajupalem, Dist. Warrangal	1979	4.40
7.	Victoria Hospital, Dichaplli, Distt. Nizamabad	1915	29.56
8.	Bethaseda Leprosy Hospital PB No. 13, Narsapur	1923	19.10
9.	Philadelphia Leprosy Hospital, Salur-532391 Dist. Vijianagaram	1966	27.00
10.	The Leprosy Mission Hospital Voluntary Organisation Dist. Vijianagaram-531230	1913	10.00
11.	Greater Visakha Leprosy Treatment and Health Education Scheme, PB No. 180, 21-1-2 A.V.N College Road, Visakhapatnam-530001	1975	8.4
12.	Emmaus-Swiss Leprosy Project, Lalamaner, Dist. Chittoor-517424	1977	16.97

(Contd.)

* Source: *Voluntary organisations in Leprosy Eradication*, Leprosy Division, Directorate General of Health Services, Government of India, New Delhi, 1988, 54p.

1.	2	3	4
13.	Vimukti Leprosy Relief Association, Kakinada, Dist. East Godavari-533003	1976	14.00
14.	Gram Nava Nirman Samithi, Baghlingampally, Hyderabad-500044	1974	3.00
15.	Sivananda Rehabilitation Home, Hyderabad-500016	1958	31.72
	BIHAR		
16.	Bharat Sevashram Sangha, Leprosy Control & Rural Welfare Services, Jamshedpur	1983	8.83
17.	Claver Social Welfare Centre, Saraikela, Dist. Singhbhum	1983	3.54
18.	*Gram Nirman Mandal Kushta Sewa Samiti, Kapasia, Kawakal, Nawadah	1962	1.36
19.	Gandhi Kusht Nivaran Pratisthan, Akhlaspur, Babua, Dist. Rohtas	1960	7.72
20.	*Nav Jagrat Manav Samaj, Vikas Kutir, Kharkai Road, Jamshedpur	1981	25.00
21.	Rajendra Sevashram, Anugarh Nagar, Mairwa, Dist. Siwan	1953	45.00
22.	Santhal Paharia Seva Mandal, Deoghar	1936	80.30
23.	Singhbhum Navjivan Niketan, Ghatsila, Singhbhum	1976	2.00
24.	TLM Saldoha Leprosy Hospital, Saldoha, Dist. Dumka	1922	8.20
25.	Vanvasi Seva Kendra, Kusta Nivaran Samiti, Adhaura, Dist. Rohtas	1979	2.50
26.	Wazir Ganj Leprosy Control Programme, BAM India, Gaya	1979	3.65
27.	Mahatma Gandhi Kusht Sevashram, Raniganj, Dist. Gaya	1979	0.73
28.	Damian Social Welfare Centre, PB No. 47, Gandhi Bhavan, Dhanbad	1964	69.00
	DELHI		
29.	*Coordinated Agency for Leprosy Welfare, Delhi	1986	—
30.	*Kusht Rogi Seva Samiti, Delhi	1963	0.11
31.	*Skin Institute and School of Dermatology, Greater Kailash-1, New Delhi	1966	25.00
	GUJARAT		
32.	*Baroda Distt. Anti-Leprosy Association, Baroda	1966	0.78
33.	Shram Mandir Trust, Singhrot, Baroda	1972	25.00

(Contd.)

1.	2	3	4
KARNATAKA			
34.	Bijapur Leprosy and Community Welfare Centre, Bijapur	1981	4.61
35.	Leprosy Control Project, CSI Hospital, Colonel Hill Road, Bangalore	1978	2.72
36.	*Hind Kusht Nivaran Singh Dakshina Kannada Distt. Branch, Falnir, Mangalore	1951	4.79
37.	Janta Trust, Yadgiri, Distt. Gulbarga	1981	1.00
38.	Katharina Kasper Leprosy Control Scheme, No. 16, Hutchins Road, Bangalore	1978	2.00
39.	Rural Health Centre, Kondajji, Dist. Chitradurga	1982	6.10
40.	St. Joseph's Leprosy Hospital, Unit of Fr. Muller's Charitable Institutions, PO Kankanadi, Mangalore	1897	13.00
41.	Sumanahalli Leprosy Project, 99, Old St. Mary's Seminary Residency Road, Bangalore	1977	10.64
42.	The Hubli Hospital for the Handicapped, PB 54, Hubli, Dharund	1970	18.36
43.	Velemegna Golekhana, Bidar, (Velemegne Hospital)	1968	NA
KERALA			
44.	Cochin Urban Leprosy Treatment & Education Scheme, Cochin	1980	5.37
45.	Damien Leprosy Institute, Ayyappankavu, Trichur Dist.	1954	14.83
46.	*International Medical Association Kerala, Ernakulam Shenoy Road, Cochin	1971	1.66
47.	Marthimothens Memorial Health & Leprosy Centre, Tathamangalam, Dist. Palghat	1982	NA
48.	Poor Leprosy Hospital, Green Gardens, Shertalley, Dist. Alleppey	1942	10.96
49.	St. Francis Leprosy Centre, Thankey Junction, Kalavamkodam, Sheretallai, Distt. Alleppey	1963	2.20
50.	St. Johns Leprosy Control & Rehabilitation, Pirappencod, Trivandrum	1964	850
51.	Paul Chittilaphilly Memorial Leprosy Eradication Project Kalladakode, Dist. Palghat	1987	NA
52.	Snehaniketan Social Centre Pattuvam, Dist. Cannanore	1981	3.00

(Contd.)

1.	2	3	4
53.	St. Martin De Porres Hospital, Cherukunnu, Dist. Cannanore	1970	5.00
	MAHARASHTRA		
54.	*Acwozn Leprosy Hospital, Wadala Bombay	1890	40.00
55.	Hathomthwaite Memorial Leprosy Services, Kagal, Marwanless Hospital, Kolhapur	1981	5.50
56.	Hemakasa. Ashok Vans, Chandrapur	1951	—
57.	Kushtarog Nivaran Samiti, Shantivan, Nere Tal-Panvel	1981	14.65
58.	* Lokbiradari Project	1973	—
59.	*Marathwada Lokseva Mandal Village Nerli, Nanded	1979	3.00
60.	Maharogi Sewa Samiti, Anandavan, Warora, Dist. Chandrapur	1951	156.87
61.	Maharogi Sewa Samiti, Manohar Dham, Dattapur, Wardha	1936	20.60
62.	*Poona District Leprosy Committee, 2nd Floor, Flat No. 35, 2-A, Moledina Road, Pune-411001 (Units at Pune & Solapur)	1956	136.20
63.	*Somnath Project,	1967	—
64.	Shri Gurudeo Kushta Seva Mandir, Amla, Dist. Amaravati	1956	0.45
65.	The Society for Eradication of Leprosy, Bombay House 24, Homi Mody Street, Bombay	1978	1.90
66.	Udyog Dham, Badrikashram, Talegaon general Hospital, Pune	1978	5.50
67.	* Urban Leprosy Centre, III & IV, Kolhapur	1981	0.32
68.	Vadala Leprosy Control & Gorapur Rehabilitation Project, Vadala, Dist. Ahmednagar	1957	2.96
69.	Vidarbha Maharogi Sewa Mandal, Tapovan, Amaravati	1950	142.00
70.	Richardson Leprosy Hospital, Miraj, Dist. Sangli	1896	14.20
71.	Mahatma Fule Kushtrog Nivaran Samiti, Pardi, Nagpur	1972	3.20
72.	Rural Comprehensive Health Scheme, 510, Sadashiv Peth, Pune	1981	2.66
73.	Dr. Bandorawalla Leprosy Hospital, Kondhawa, Pune	1956	50.00
74.	Ahmednagar District, Leprosy Relief Association, Ahmednagar	1979	1.45
75.	Pune Urban Leprosy Investigation Centre, "Manisha" 2nd Floor, Flat No. 35, 2-A, Moledina Road, Pune	1975	5.46

(Contd.)

1.	2	3	4
76.	Solapur Comprehensive Leprosy Project, 142A, Bhide Colony, Solapur	1980	4.73
77.	Kusht Nivaran Davakhana, Vadoli-Talasari, Dist. Thana	1957	2.87
78.	Maharashtra Lokahita Seva Mandal, St. Francis Avenue, Santacruz (W), Bombay	1976	12.41
79.	Eduljee Framjee Albless, Leprosy Home, Trombay, Bombay	1885	3.00
80.	Assisi Sevasadan Hospital, Nagepalli, Distt. Sadehiroli, Gadchiroli	1974	0.74
81.	International Leprosy Union, 90, CASP Pune Unit, 16/6, Raghudurg Apartment, Erandavana, Pune	1987	0.50
82.	Rural Integrated Health Scheme, Kargat, Dist. Raigad	1982	4.28
83.	Bombay Leprosy Project, Vidnyan Bhavan, 11VN Purav Marg, Sion-Chunabhatti, Bombay	1976	22.46
84.	Shakti Brahmashram, C/o JES College, Jalna	1979	0.25
85.	Norwegian Free Evangelical Mission India, PB No. 10, Chopda, Distt. Jalgaon	1951	25.00
	MADHYA PRADESH		
86.	Pushpa Hospital, Dalli-Rajhara, Dist. Durg	1984	2.86
87.	*Shantipur Leprosy Hospital PB No. 64, PO Dhamtari, Raipur	1922	2.99
88.	The Leprosy Mission Voluntary SET Programme, Leprosy Hospital & Home, Baitalpur, Dist Bilaspur	1968	2.68
	ORISSA		
89.	*Divya Jivan Arogya Kendra, Khurda Road, Puri	1976	0.05
90.	Mayurbhanj Leprosy Home, Baripada, Mayurbhanj	1903	2.50
91.	Puri Urban Leprosy Project, Duttatola, Puri	1981	3.98
92.	Anantha Annadana Kendra and Databya Chikitsalaya, Prajabandhu Ashra, Aska, Ganjam Dist.	1981	1.00
93.	Hind Kusht Nivaran Sangh, Red Cross Bhavan, Bhubaneshwar	1950	52.17
94.	Assisi Leprosy Hospital Tamilnadu Centre, Talavadi, Dist. Periyar	1970	5.74
95.	*C.S.I. Medical & Leprosy Centres, Vandavasi	1980	—
96.	Christian Fellowship Community Health Centre, Ambilikkai, Dist. Anna	1966	3.84
97.	Christian Hospital, Madarapakkam	1952	3.40

(Contd.)

1.	2	3	4
98.	**Dinabandhu Medical Mission, RK Pet., Chingalpattu	1962	0.94
99.	Holy Family Hansenorium, Fathima Nagar, Tiruchirapalli	1955	8.29
100.	*I.E.L.C. Leprosy Control Project Mission Compound, Ambur Dist. North Arcot	1975	3.58
101.	Kasturba Kustha Nivaran Nilayam, Malavanthangal, Kandachipuram	1946	7.22
102.	Leprosy Relief Rural Centre, Settipatty, Salem	1956	20.00
103.	Rawttakuppam Hemerjick Rural Centre, Auroville, Dist. South Arcot	1960	11.00
104.	St. Thomas Hospital & Leprosy Centre, Chettupattu, Distt. North Arcot	1960	32.50
105.	The Society of Sacred Heart Leprosy Centre, Salakottai, Kumbakonam, Dist. Thanjavur	1963	41.00
106.	Shieffelin Leprosy Research & Training Centre, Karigiri, Dist. North Arcot	1955	69.42
107.	The Kumbakonam Hindu Mission Hospital, 13, Mutt Street, Kumbakonam	1977	7.58
108.	Worth Trust, 41, Tirrukallum Road, Katpadi, North Arcot	1963	19.00
109.	The Leprosy Voluntary SET Centre, The Leprosy Mission, Vadathora Salur, Tiyagadrug, Dist. South Arcot	1925	13.42
110.	GREMALTES Referral Hospital & Leprosy Centre Shenoinagar, Madras	1971	27.47
111.	German Leprosy Relief Association, Shenoinagar, Madras	1969	316.33
112.	Leprosy Relief Work, Emmaus-Switzerland, 4 Gajapathy Street, Shenoynagar, Madras	1969	134.42
113.	Kasturba Kusht Nivaran Nilayam, Kanchipuram	1945	7.22
114.	Arogya Agam, Anndipatty, Periakulam Taluk, Dist. Madurai	1963	5.00
115.	CHAD Hospital, Leprosy Control Programme, Christian Medical College & Hospital, Vellore, Dist. North Arcot	1970	4.96
116.	The Voluntary Health Services, Adyar, Madras	1958	57.00
117.	Damien Leprosy Control Centre, Diwaniangar, Nilakottai, Dist. Anna	1969	5.14
118.	Poorna Sukha Leprosy Project, St. Joseph Hospital, Dindigal, Dist. Anna	1959	4.22
119	St. Mary's Leprosy Centre, Arisipalayam, Salem	1961	5.00
120.	Hindu Mission Hospital, 36, GST Road, Tambaram, Madras	1984	NA

(Contd.)

1.	2	3	4
121.	The Leprosy Mission Hospital, Dayapuram, Mamamadurai	1962	3.53
122.	St. Joseph's Leprosy Hospital, Arokkla Puram, Dist. Tuticorin	—	NA
123.	Jothi Nilayam Rural Hospital & Leprosy Control Centre, GSI, Vellore, Muttathur, Dist. South Arcot	1941	2.97
	UTTAR PRADESH		
124.	St. Joseph's Hospital, 372, Civil Lines, Roorkee, Distt. Saharanpur	1977	0.56
125.	B.R.D. Kustha Sevashram, Deoria	1952	4.50
126.	* Kashi Kustha Sevashram Sangh, Ashapur, Sarnath, Varanasi	1961	1.63
127.	Poorvanchal Seva Sansthan, Deoria	1978	1.86
128.	Jahangir Memorial Charitable Hospital, 558, Bahadur Ganj, Allahabad	1979	15.00
129.	The Leprosy Mission, Chandag, Dist. Pithoragarh	1981	NA
130.	Sanjaya Gandhi Seva Sansthan, Deoria	1983	2.28
131.	Leprosy Hospital & Home, Karbala, Dist. Almora	1854	4.00
132.	Kanpur Kusht Nivaran Sansthan, Nawab Ganj, Kanpur	1984	0.05
133.	Prem Sewa Hospital, Utrania, Dist. Gonda	1960	13.6
	WEST BENGAL		
134.	Adra Leprosy Project, Adra, Purulia Dist.	1986	4.23
135.	* Garden Reach Community Health Programme, BAM India, Paharpur Road, Gardenreach, Calcutta	—	—
136.	Greater Calcutta Leprosy Treatment & Health Education Scheme, 35/1/A Old Ballygunge, 1st Lane, Calcutta	1975	10.13
137.	Jhargram Leprosy Project, (GLRA) Midnapur Jhargram	1977	6.19
138.	*Leprosy Field Research Unit, Jhalda	1965	4.90
139.	Mahakuma Kushta Nibarani Samiti, Gidni, Dist. Midnapur	1970	2.50
140.	*St. Bernadettis Dispensary, Bhimghar, Shahabad, Dist. Darjeeling	1969	0.4
141.	St. Vincent De paul Leprosy Clinic, Hatighisa, Dist. Darjeeling	1970	0.22
142.	The Leprosy Mission, Bankura Leprosy Control Programme & Hospital, Innbedia, Dist. Bankura	1902	11.73

(Contd.)

1.	2	3	4
143.	Calcutta Urban Service, 16, Sudder Street, Calcutta	1969	3.40
144.	Grameen Sarbatmak Kalyan Kendra, 68, Lenin Sarani, Calcutta	1975	NA
	PONDICHERY		
145.	Raoul Follereau Foundation, No. 2, Curcouf Street, Pondichery	1983	13.00
	SEVERAL STATES		
146.	*Damien Foundation in India (6 field centres besides 16 sponsored centres)	1978	170.00
147.	Gandhi Memorial Leprosy Foundation, Hindnagar, Wardha (Maharashtra)	1951	35.92
148.	* German Leprosy Relief Association, 4, Gajapathi Street, Shenoy Nagar, Madras (T.N.)	1969	400.00
149.	* Leprosy Relief Work, Emmaus, Switzerland 4, Gajapathi St., Shenoy Street, Madras (T.N.)		
150.	* The Leprosy Mission, Delhi (32 own & 37 aided centres)	–	374.94
151.	* Hind Kusht Nivaran Sangha	1950	40.00
	Total		3298.31

* The figures are based on the report upto March, 1986.

** Has been taken over by Government of Tamil Nadu in the year 1986-87.

NA Not Available.

TABLE A24.2: Survey, Education and Treatment (SET) Activities of Voluntary Organisations (As on 1-4-1987)

Sl. No.	Name of Voluntary Organisation	Population covered (in lakh)	Prevalence rate/ 1000	Case detected on record	Case under treatment	Cases discharged
(1)	(2)	(3)	(4)	(5)	(6)	(7)
	ANDHRA PRADESH					
1.	*Assist Sisters of Assisi Nagar, Komkepudi Via-Pedana, Krishna Dist.	1.79	9.6	1735	1510	178
2.	Comprehensive Health Care Unit, Parvatipuram, Vizianagaram Dist.	0.60	4.2	253	253	1128
3.	Greater Tenali Leprosy Treatment & Health Education Scheme Gandhi nagar, Tenali	1.10	18.7	2057	1417	640
4.	Asha Niketan, Kavali, Nellore Distt.	0.55	10.7	587	333	162
5.	H.K.N.S. Jammikunta, Karimnagar Dist.	2.69	11.7	3153	3153	854
6.	Victoria Hospital, Dichpalli, Nizamabad Dist.	1.18	0.8	91	91	132
7.	Bethesda Leprosy Hospital, PB No. 13, Narsapur,	1.89	6.4	1211	964	724
8.	Philadelphia Leprosy Hospital, Salur, Vizianagaram Distt.	1.84	1.7	306	306	2058
9.	The Leprosy Mission Voluntary Organization, Chelluru, Dist. Vizianagaram	2.38	2.9	692	692	5398
10.	Grama Nava Nirman Samithi, Baghlingampally, Hyderabad	3.13	0.9	282	273	Nil
11.	Vimukti Leprosy Relief Association, Kakinada, Dist. East Godavari	1.83	8.7	1589	1589	272
12.	Sivananda Rehabilitation Home, Hyderabad	3.65	9.4	3413	3290	423

(Contd.)

(1)	(2)	(3)	(4)	(5)	(6)	(7)
BIHAR						
13.	Bharat Sevashram Sangha Leprosy Control & Rural Welfare Services, Jamshedpur	8.94	17.0	15201	10793	1500
14.	Claver Social Welfare Centre, Sarakela, Singhbhum	2.00	20.7	4163	3094	1894
15.	Gandhi Kusht Nivaran Pratisthan, Akhlaspur, Distt. Rohtas	12.60	9.3	11758	10108	10003
16.	Gram Nirman Mandal Kusht Sews Samiti, Kapasia, Nawadah	2.27	0.3	79	77	66
17.	Rajendra Sevashram, Anugrah Nagar Mairwa, Siwan Distt.	22.16	8.8	19446	16637	5301
18.	Santhal Paharia Seva Mandal, Deoghar,	10.09	12.3	12459	5683	4093
19.	TLM Saldoha Leprosy Hospital, Sadoha, Distt. Dumka	1.38	8.4	11.62	1130	364
20.	Singhbhum Navjeevan Niketan, Ghatsila, Singhbhum	2.04	20.1	4101	3221	115
21.	V.S.K. Kusht Nivaran Samiti, Adhaura, Rothas Distt.	0.93	8.0	744	744	50
22.	Wazir Ganj Leprosy Control Programme, BAM India, Gaya	0.95	48.9	4644	4280	164
23.	Damien Social Welfare Centre, PB No. 47, Gandhi Bhavan, Dhanbad,	13.15	15.4	20267	17002	10692
24.	Mahatma Gandhi Kusht Sevashram, Raniganj, Dist. Gaya	1.04	5.0	517	380	NA
DELHI						
25.	*Coordinated Agency for Leprosy Welfare, Delhi	–	–	4	4	–
26.	*Skin Institute & School of Dermatology, GK.I, New Delhi	–	–	1000	1000	–
GUJARAT						
27.	Shram Mandir Trust Sindhorot, Baroda	1.4	9.53	472	438	965
28.	*Baroda District Anti-Leprosy Association, Baroda	1.08	4.2	452	452	599

(Contd.)

(1)	(2)	(3)	(4)	(5)	(6)	(7)
KARNATAKA						
29.	*Bijapur Leprosy and Community Welfare Centre, Bijapur	0.84	6.1	515	515	144
30.	Leprosy Control Project, CSI Hospital, 2, Colonel Hill Road, Bangalore	1.65	2.4	400	213	221
31.	*H.K.N.S. Dakshina Kannada, Mangalore	6.44	10.7	6901	6901	3841
32.	Janta Trust, Yadgir, Gulbarga	1.03	8.6	888	888	500
33.	Kathrina Kesper Leprosy Control Scheme Bangalore	NA	–	571	376	883
34.	Rural Health Centre, Kondajji, Chitradurga	2.43	10.3	2491	610	1881
35.	Sumanahalli Society, Old St. Mary's Seminary Building Bangalore	3.87	1.7	669	628	545
36.	Hubli Hospital for Handicapped Hubli	3.32	1.6	547	430	391
37.	Velemegna Golkhana, Bidar	0.24	17.6	423	423	137
38.	St. Joseph's Leprosy Hospital, Kankandy, Mangalore	0.55	27.8	1530	1507	767
KERALA						
39.	Cochin Urban Leprosy Treatment & Education Scheme, Cochin	2.61	4.5	1169	1042	832
40.	Damien Leprosy Institute Ayyappan Kavu, Trichur Distt.	1.05	5.0	522	509	751
41.	*International Medical Association Ernakulam, Shenoy Road, Cochin	0.58	7.0	404	391	303
42.	Marthimothens Memorial Health & Leprosy Centre, Tathamangalam, Palghat Distt.	2.03	6.4	1309	1135	280
43.	Poor Leprosy Hospital, Green, Gardens, Shertalley, Alleppy Distt.	1.12	4.6	513	479	405
44.	Francis Leprosy Centre Shertalley, Alleppy Distt.	1.09	1.8	200	181	750

(Contd.)

(1)	(2)	(3)	(4)	(5)	(6)	(7)
45.	St. John's Leprosy Control & Rahabilitation, Pirappencod, Trivandrum	0.48	51.5	2474	2117	612
46.	St. Martin De Porres Hospital, Cherukunnu, Cannanore Distt.	1.00	4.5	451	438	12
47.	Snehaniketan Social Centre, Pattuvam, Cannanore Dist.	1.00	2.9	287	238	147
48.	Paul Chittilapilly Memorial Leprosy Eradication Project, Kalladikode, Palghat Distt.	0.15	4.3	65	49	3
	MADHYA PRADESH					
49.	Pushpa Hospital, Dalli-Rajhara, Durg, Distt.	1.23	4.1	502	486	NA
50.	The Leprosy Mission, Voluntary SET Programme, Chandkhuri Leprosy Hospital & Home, Baitalpur, Bilaspur Dist.	1.16	3.1	363	363	650
	MAHARASHTRA					
51.	* Acworth Leprosy Hospital Wadala Bombay	15.00	16.7	25000	20000	5000
52.	* Kusthrog Nivaran Samiti, Santivan, Raigad	1.72	9.4	1611	1274	694
53.	* Lokbiradari Project	—	—	25	25	—
54.	* Marathwada Loksewa Mandal Nerli, Nanded	1.82	3.2	588	588	198
55.	Maha Rogi Sewa Samiti, Manohar Dham, Dattapur, Wardha	0.71	1.9	136	136	981
56.	* Poona District Leprosy Committee, 2nd Floor, Flat No. 35-2A Moledina, Pune	5.00	15.2	7587	7586	1936
57.	Shri Gurudeo Kustha Seva Mandir, Amla, Vishveshwar, Amravati Distt.	0.26	2.4	63	63	475
58.	Society for Eradication of Leprosy, Bombay House, 24-Homi Mody Street, Bombay	0.35	16.4	574	522	16
59.	* Somnath Project	—	—	500	500	—
60.	* Urban Leprosy Centre III & IV. Kolhapur	0.97	6.0	574	566	4

(Contd.)

(1)	(2)	(3)	(4)	(5)	(6)	(7)
61.	Vadala Leprosy Control & Gorapur Rehabilitation Project, Vadala Mission, Ahmednagar	2.64	4.0	1058	1047	452
62.	Richardson Leprosy Hospital, Miraj, Sangli Distt.	2.39	2.2	531	531	2146
63.	Rural Comprehensive Health Scheme, 510, Sadashiv Peth, Pune	1.01	3.3	332	319	353
64.	Ahmednagar Distt. Leprosy Relief Association, Satane Wade, Ahmednagar	2.57	3.7	937	937	244
65.	Hathornthwaite Memorial Leprosy Services, Kagal, Kolhapur	2.37	7.4	1750	1705	1250
66.	Rural Integrated Health Scheme, Karjat, Raigad Distt.	1.48	6.7	992	688	1158
67.	Maharashtra Likahita Seva mandal, St. Francis Avenue, Santacruz (W), Bombay	6.69	15.0	10036	5257	3224
68.	Kusht Nivaran Davakhana, Vadoli-Talasari PO. Thana Distt.	1.06	6.4	678	678	617
69.	Solapur Comprehensive Leprosy Project, Bhide Colony, Solapur	3.18	6.3	2014	1922	1132
70.	Pune Urban Leprosy Investigation Centre, "Manisha", 2nd Floor, Flat No. 35, 2-A, Moledina Road, Pune	4.69	6.2	2913	1777	1697
71.	Assisi Sevasadan Hospital, Nagepalli, Gadchiroli Distt.	0.60	18.4	1104	208	919
72.	Bombay Leprosy Project, Vidnyan Bhavan, II VN Purav Marg, Sion-Chunabhatti, Bombay	NA	—	7836	7836	1299
73.	Shaktibrahmashram, C/o JES College, Jalna	0.62	3.1	191	183	60
74.	Norwegian Free Evangelical Mission India, PB No. 10, Chopda Jalgaon Dist.	NA	—	37	37	NA
75.	Kusharog Nivaran Samiti, Santivan, Post, Nere, Tal-Panvel	1.61	7.3	1168	1075	709

(Contd.)

(1)	(2)	(3)	(4)	(5)	(6)	(7)
ORISSA						
76.	* Divya Jiwan Arogya Kendra, Khura Road, Puri	0.42	16.7	700	472	70
77.	Puri Urban Leprosy Project, Sadar Thana Lane, Puri	1.16	19.4	2254	2020	403
TAMIL NADU						
78.	Assisi Leprosy Hospital Centre, Talavadi, Distt. Periyar	0.75	13.6	1020	1020	454
79.	*C.S.I. Medical Leprosy Centre, Vanda Vasi	1.39	17.5	2426	2002	1933
80.	Christian Fellowship Community Health Centre, Ambilikkai, Anna Dist.	1.22	12.3	1503	1246	89
81.	Christian Hospital, Madarapakkam	0.35	16.1	564	349	154
82.	** Dinbandhu Medical Mission R.K. Pet, Chingalpur	1.65	10.4	1715	1715	—
83.	Holy Family Hansenorium, Fathimanagar, Tiruchirapally	2.35	8.0	1891	1804	2772
84.	* I.E.L.C. Leprosy Control Project, Mission Compound, Ambur, North Arcot	1.61	5.9	953	689	330
85.	Kasturba Kushtha Nivaran Nilayam, Malayanthangal, Kandachipuram	2.41	6.6	1590	1564	8059
86.	* Leprosy Relief Rural Centre, Chettipatti	5.0	44.3	22176	4141	9760
87.	Rawtakuppam Hemerjick Rural Centre, Auroville, South Arcot-605101	2.50	8.6	2156	2156	10246
88.	Schieffin Leprosy Research & Training Centre, Karigiri, North Arcot Distt.	6.40	7.5	4806	4109	12453
89.	St. Thomas Hospital and Leprosy Centre, Chettupattu, North Arcot Distt.	3.50	4.8	1688	1688	12595
90.	The Kumbakonam Hindu Mission Hospital, 13, Mutt Street, Kumbakonam	10.75	11.6	12506	10538	6628
91.	The Leprosy Mission Hospital, Dayapuram, Mamamadurai	2.09	2.4	501	395	1643

(Contd.)

(1)	(2)	(3)	(4)	(5)	(6)	(7)
92.	Jothy Nilayam Rural Hospital & Leprosy Control Centre Muttathur, South Arcot, Dist.	1.16	19.6	2277	1663	362
93.	St. Joseph's Leprosy Hospital, Arokkiapuram, Dist. Tuticorin	0.39	69.1	2694	1716	1430
94.	The Leprosy Voluntary SET Centre, Leprosy Mission, Vadathorasalur, Tiyagadrug, South Arcot Distt.	1.14	3.3	372	372	2375
95.	GREMLTES Referral Hospital & Leprosy Centre, 5, Gajapathy St. Shenoyanagar, Madras	17.00	3.5	5887	4675	11929
96.	Arogya Agam, Aundipatty, Periakulam Tq., Madurai Distt.	1.71	5.5	944	878	2621
97.	CHAD Hospital, Leprosy Control Programme, Christian Medical College, Vellore, North Arcot Dist.	2.10	9.3	1943	1843	3905
98,	The Voluntary Health Service, Adyar, Madras	1.37	12.4	1692	1692	526
99.	Damien Leprosy Control Centre, Diravianagar, Nilakottai, Anna Dist.	1.59	13.7	2171	1965	1525
100.	Leprosy Relief Rural Centre, Settpatty, Omlaur, Salem Dist.	2.53	31.6	7991	2053	5014
101.	Poorna Sukha Leprosy Project, St. Joseph Hospital, Dindigul, Ann Dist.	2.04	4.9	1002	827	1704
102.	St. Mary's Leprosy Centre, Arisipalayam, Salem	2.57	15.7	4031	3361	2244
103.	Hindu Mission Hospital 36, GST Road, Madras	2.30	10.3	2378	1901	975
	UTTAR PRADESH					
104.	St. Joseph's Hospital, 372, Civil Lines, Roorkee Dist. Saharanpur	1.17	0.9	103	103	42
105	B.R.D. Kustha Sevashram, Deoria	2.47	6.4	1582	1582	1530
106	* Kashi Kusht Seva Sangha, Sarnath, Varanasi	6.0	4.9	2957	1243	26
107.	Poorvanchal Sevasansthan, Deoria	2.30	7.6	1742	1723	650

(Contd.)

(1)	(2)	(3)	(4)	(5)	(6)	(7)
108.	Jahangir Memorial Charitable Hospital, 558, Bahadur Ganj, Allahabad	1.69	7.0	1184	1141	22
109.	The Leprosy Mission, Changad, Dist. Pithoragarh	1.70	7.0	1192	856	154
110.	Sanjaya Gandhi Seva Sansthan, Deoria	2.49	6.5	1615	946	471
111.	Kanpur Kusht Nivaran Sansthan, Nawab Ganj, Kanpur	NA	—	163	163	132
112.	Prem Sewa Hospital, Utraula, Gonda Dist.	NA	—	12523	2851	670
113.	Leprosy Hospital & Home, Karbala, Almora	NA	—	441	314	137
WEST BENGAL						
114.	Adra Leprosy Project, Adra, Purulia Distt.	1.04	26.8	2786	2323	968
115.	Calcutta Urban Service, 16, Calcutta	5.06	2.02	1024	768	3
116.	* Garden Reach Community Health Programme, BAM India, Paharpur Road, Calcutta	3.50	3.8	1332	861	1627
117.	Greater Calcutta Leprosy Treatment & Health Education Scheme 35/1/A, Old Ballygunge, Calcutta	6.62	1.5	1006	852	2145
118.	Jhargram Leprosy Project (GLRA), Jhargram, Midnapore Dist.	1.81	24.3	4401	3810	1578
119.	* Leprosy Field Research Unit, Jhalda	0.20	—	—	—	—
120.	* St. Bernadettis Dispensary Bhimghar, Shahabad, Darjeeling	0.40	72.2	2890	2423	245
121.	Mahakuma Kusht Nibaran Samiti, Gidni, Midnapore Dist.	2.10	15.9	3331	2843	227
122.	St. Vincent De Paul Leprosy Clinic, Hatizhisa, Darjeeling Dist.	0.15	21.9	329	325	142
123.	The Leprosy Mission, Bankura Leprosy Control Programme & Hospital, Junbedia, Bankura Dist.	3.80	7.7	2941	2781	5000

(Contd.)

(1)	(2)	(3)	(4)	(5)	(6)	(7)
124.	Grameen Sarbatmar Kalyan Kendra, 68, Lenin Sarani, Calcutta	1.93	2.4	471	306	NA
PONDICHERRY						
125.	Raoul Fallerean Foundation No. 2, Surcouf Street, Pondicherry					
VOLUNTARY ORGANISATIONS IN MORE THAN ONE STATE		—	—	136	136	20
126.	* Damien Foundation in India (6 field centres beside 16 sponsored centres)	12.00	18.3	21989	21989	3958
127.	Gandhi Memorial Leprosy Foundation, Hindi Nagar, Wardha (Maharashtra)	4.68	9.8	4580	4580	13012
128.	German Leprosy Relief Association, 4, Gajapathy St. Shenoyanagar, Madras, TN	178.36	8.9	159118	99737	51704
129.	** HKNS Delhi	7.96	7.0	5557	4230	678
130.	Leprosy Relief Work, Emmaus-Switzerland, 4, Gajapathy St. (X) Shenoy Nagar Madras	38.98	10.0	39128	31254	14054
131.	** The Leprosy Mission, Delhi (32 own & 37 aided)	48.77	42.0	205096	205096	1887
	Total	607.9	1.27	774824	623951	289695

* The figures are based on the report upto March, 1986.

** Has been taken over by Government of Tamil Nadu in the year 1986-87.

NA Not Available

TABLE A24.3: Name of Voluntary Organisations with Leprosy Hospital/Homes/ Rehabilitation Activities

Sl. No.	Name of voluntary organisation	No. of beds	No. of patients rehabilitated as on 1.4.87	
			Medical	Vocational
(1)	(2)	(3)	(4)	(5)
	ANDHRA PRADESH			
1.	Greater Tenali Leprosy Treatment & Health Education Scheme, Gandhinagar, Tenali	—	—	86
2.	Asha Niketan Health Centre, Vengal Rao Nagar, Kavali	6	—	—
3.	Hind Kushtha Nivaran Sangha, Jammikunta, Karimnagar Distt.	25	15	85
4.	* St. Joseph Leprosy Rehabilitation Centre, PO Thimmaraju palem, Dist. Warangal	80	—	77
5.	Victoria Hospital, Dichpalli, Distt. Nizamabad	100	5	3
6.	Bethesda Leprosy Hospital, PB No. 13, Narsapur	150	(445)	45
7.	Philadelphia Leprosy Hospital, Salur, Vizianagram Distt.	145	—	—
8.	The Leprosy Mission Voluntary organization, Chelluru, Vizianagaram Dist.	40	—	2
9.	Grama Nava Nirman Samithi, Baghlingampally, Hyderabad	NA	6	20
10.	Vimukti Leprosy Relief Association, Kakinada, East Godavari Distt.	10	13	100
11.	Sivananda Rehabilitation Home, Hyderabad	120	63	202
12.	Greater Visakha Leprosy Treatment & Health Education Scheme, PB No. 180, Visakhapatnam	20	15	107
13.	Emmaus-Swiss Leprosy Project, Palamaner, Distt. Chittoor	35	44	26

(Contd.)

(1)	(2)	(3)	(4)	(5)
BIHAR				
14.	Bharat Sevashram Sangha Leprosy Control & Welfare Services, Jamshedpur	60	9	77
15.	Claver Social Welfare Centre, Saraikela, Singhbhum	—	(152)	—
16.	Gandh Kushtha Nivaran Pratisthan Akhlaspur, Distt. Rohtas	50	NA	NA
17.	** Gram Nirman Mandal, Kushtha Seva Samiti, Kapasia, Nevadan	40	40	—
18.	** Nivjagrat Manav Samaj Nidhi, Jamshedpur, Bihar	31	25	25
19.	Rajendra Sevashra, Anugrah Nagar, Manwa, Siwan Distt.	200	30	700
20.	TLM Sadoha Leprosy Hospital, Saldoha Distt. Dumka	60	—	—
21.	Singhbhum Navjiwan Niketan, Moubhandar, Ghatsila, Singhbhum	NA	6	Nil
22.	Santhal Paharia Seva Mandal, Deoghar	140	(4093)	7
23.	Vanvasi Seva Kendra, Kushta Nivaran Samiti, Adhaura, Distt. Rohtas	10	NA	NA
24.	Damien Social Welfare Centre, PB No. 47, Dhanbad Gandhi Bhavan	210	29	161
DELHI				
25.	* Coordinated Agency for Leprosy Welfare, Delhi	—	—	12
26.	* Skin Institute & School of Dermatalogy, G.K.I. New Delhi	30	—	35
GUJARAT				
27.	Shram Mandir Trust, Sindhrot, Baroda	70	(280)	500
KARNATAKA				
28.	*H.K.N.S. Dakshina Kannada, Mangalore-1	—	5	3

(Contd.)

(1)	(2)	(3)	(4)	(5)
29.	Hubli Hospital for the Handicapped PB 54, Hubli	60	NA	166
30.	Rural Health Centre, Kondajji, Chitradurga, Distt.	20	NA	NA
31.	Sumanhal Society, No. 99, Old St. Mary's Seminary Residency Bldg, Bangalore	7	–	–
32.	St. Joseph's Leprosy Hospital, Kankanady Mangalore	140	(500)	155
33.	Velemegna Golkhana Bidar	155	(160)	20
34.	Leprosy Control Project, CSI Hospital 2, Colonel Hill Road, Bangalore	10	NA	NA
KERALA				
35.	Cochin Uman Leprosy Treatment & Education Scheme, Cochin-6	NA	134	11
36.	Damien Leprosy Institute, Ayyappan Kavu, Trichur	195	3	4
37.	Marthimomens Memorial Health & Leprosy Centre, Tathamanpalam, Palghat Dist.	13	–	–
38.	Poor Leprosy Hospital, Green Gardens, Shertalley, Alleppey Distt.	200	–	–
39.	St. Francis Leprosy Centre, Thanky Junction, Kalavamkodam, Snertalli, Distt. Alleppey	12	1050	–
40.	St. John's Leprosy Control & Rehabilitation, Pirappencod, Trivandrum	40	4	8
41.	St. Martin Deporres Hospital, Cherukunnu, Distt. Cannanore	73	–	–
42.	Snehaniketan Social Centre, Pattuvam, Distt. Cannanore	15	NA	NA
MAHARASHTRA				
43.	* Adworth Leprosy Hospital, Wadala, Bombay	500	150	350
44.	Shri Gurudeo Kushta Seva Mandir, Amla Vishveshwar, Amravati Distt.	5	–	–

(Contd.)

(1)	(2)	(3)	(4)	(5)
45.	Hathomtowaite Memorial Leprosy Services, Kagal, Kolhapur	11	2	2
46.	* Hemakasa, Ashokavana Chandrapur	100	–	–
47.	Kustha Rog Nivaran Samiti, Shantivan, PO Nera, Talpanvel	75	–	27
48.	* Marathwada Loksewa Mandal Nerli, Nanded	–	5	85
49.	Maharog Sewa Samiti, Manohar Dham, Dattapur, Wardha	850	(705)	719
50.	Maharog Seva Samiti, Warora, Chandrapur Distt.	NA	(808)	507
51.	Dr. Sancorawalla Leprosy Hospital, Poona District Leprosy Committee, Flat No. 35, 2-A Moledina Road, Pune	450	NA	NA
52.	* Udyogonam	12	–	17
53.	* Urban Leprosy Centre III & IV, Kolhapur	5	–	–
54.	Vadala Leprosy Control and Gorapur Rehabilitation Project, Vadala, Ahmedanagar Distt.	10	75	250
55.	Vidharbha Maharogi Seva Mandal, Tapovan, Amravati Distt.	150	(543)	1425
56.	Mahatma Fule Kushtrog Nivaran Samiti, Pardi, Nagpur	NA	31	30
57.	Richardson Leprosy Hospital, Miraj, Sangli Distt.	120	14	20
58.	Rural Comprehensive Health Scheme, 510, Sadashiv Peth, Pune	NA	–	–
59.	Ahmednagar Distt. Leprosy Relief Association, Ahmednagar	200	–	–
60.	Rural Integrated Health Scheme, Karjat, Distt. Raigad	NA	–	–
61.	Maharashtra Lokahite Seva Mandal, St. Francis Avenue, Santacruz (W), Bombay	112	78	153
62.	Kusht Nivaran Davakhana, Vadoli, Distt. Thana	39	–	–
63.	Solapur Comprehensive Leprosy Project, 142A, Bhide Colony, Solapur	NA	(163)	41

(Contd.)

(1)	(2)	(3)	(4)	(5)
64.	Eduljee Framjee Albless Leprosy Home, Trombay, Bombay	90	3	5
65.	Assisi Sevasadan Hospital, Nagepalli, Distt. Gadchiroli	25	–	–
66.	Bombay Leprosy Project, Vidnyan Bhavan, 11 VN, Purav Marg, Sion-Chunabhatti, Bombay	20	NA	NA
67.	Norwegian Free Evangelical Mission India, PB No. 10, Chopda, Distt. Jalgaon	45	NA	NA
	MADHYA PRADESH			
68.	Pushpa Hospital, Dalli-Rajhara, Distt. Durg	10	–	–
69.	The Leprosy Mission, voluntary SET Programme, Chandkhuri Leprosy Hospital & Home, Baitalpur, Distt. Bilaspur	175	Nil	Nil
	TAMIL NADU			
70.	Assisi Leprosy Hospital Centre, Talavadi, Distt. Periyar	9	NA	NA
71.	*C.S.I. Medical & Leprosy Centre, Vandavasi	10	12	18
72.	Christian Fellowship Community Health Centre, Ambilikkai, Distt. Anna	80	33	4
73.	Christian Hospital, Madarapakkam	40	NA	NA
74.	** Dinabandhu Medical Mission, R.K. Pet, Chingalput	–	–	50
75.	Holy Family Hansenorium, Fathimanagar, Trichurapally	100	107	195
76.	Kasturba Kustha Nivaran Nilayam, Kanchipuram	80	(4724)	3001
77.	St. Thomas Hospital & Leprosy Centre, Chettupattu	90	47	292
78.	Rawttakuppam Hemerjickx Centre, Auroville, South Arcot Distt.	30	(3000)	686

(Contd.)

(1)	(2)	(3)	(4)	(5)
79.	The Society of Sacred Heart Leprosy Centre, Kumbakonam, Tanjavur Distt.	470	–	485
80.	Schieffelin Leprosy Research & Training Centre, Karigiri, North Arcot Distt.	180	NA	237
81.	Leprosy Relief Rural Centre, Settipatty, Salem	90	(582)	60
82.	** Worth Trust, 48, New Tiruvallam Road, Katpadi, Vellore, North Arcot	30	(3000)	700
83.	St. Josephes Leprosy Hospital, Arkkiapuram Distt. Turicorin	300	NA	NA
84.	Jothi Nilayam Rural Hospital & Leprosy Control Centre, Muttathur, South Arcot Dist.	25	NA	NA
85.	The Leprosy Mission Hospital, Dayapuram, Mammadurai	70	NA	NA
86.	The Leprosy Voluntary SET Centre, The Leprosy Mission, Vadathorasalur, Tiyagadrug, Distt. South Arcot	195	8	3
87.	GREMALTES Referral Hospital & Leprosy Centre, 5, Gajapathy Street Shenoynagar, Madras	85	(355)	1442
88.	Arogya Agam, Aundipatty, Taluk Periakulam, Distt. Maduri	35	28	–
89.	Mary's Leprosy Centre, Arisipalayam, Salem	15	(1075)	–
90.	CHAD Hospital, Leprosy Control Programme, Christian Medical College & Hospital, Vellore, Distt. North Arcot	26	12	52
91.	The Voluntary Health Services, Adyar, Madras	16	–	–
92.	Damien Leprosy Control Centre, Diravianagar, Nilakottai, Distt. Anna	44	30	279
93.	Poorna Sukha Leprosy Project, St. Joseph Hospital, Dindigul, Distt. Anna	23	–	–

(Contd.)

(1)	(2)	(3)	(4)	(5)
ORISSA				
94.	Mayurbhanj Leprosy Home, PB No. 23, Baripada, Mayurbhanj	100	–	–
95.	Hind Kusht Nivaran Sangh, Red Cross Bhavan, Bhubaneswar	30	20	80
96.	Anatha Annadana Kendra and Databya Chikichalaya, Aska, Distt. Ganjam	NA	–	12
UTTAR PRADESH				
97.	BRD Kustha Sevashram Hospital, Deoria	75	15	29
98.	* Kashi Kustha Seva Sangh, Ashapur, Sarnath, Varanasi	20	31	8
99.	Poorvanchal Seva Sansthan, Deoria	10	–	–
100.	Jahangir Memorial Charitable Hospital, 558, Bahadur Ganj, Allahabad	25	–	–
101.	The Leprosy Mission, Chandog, Distt. Pithoragarh	60	–	20
102.	Leprosy Hospital & Home, Karbala, Dist. Almora	80	–	–
103.	Sanjay Gandhi Seva Sansthan, Deoria	10	–	–
104.	Prem Sewa Hospital Utraula, Distt. Gonda	11	NA	NA
WEST BENGAL				
105.	Jhargram Leprosy Project, Jhargram, Distt. Midnapore	8	25	27
106.	Mahakuma Kustha Nibarani Samiti, Gidni, Distt. Madnapore	–	94	67
107.	Calcutta Urban Service, 16, Sudder Street, Calcutta	NA	NA	NA
108.	Greater Calcutta Leprosy Treatment & Health Education Scheme, 35/1/A, Old Balygunge, 1st Lane, Calcutta	3	3	–

(Contd.)

(1)	(2)	(3)	(4)	(5)
109.	Adra Leprosy Project, Adra, Distt. Purulia	–	5	4
	VOs HAVING BRANCH IN SEVERAL STATES			
110.	* Damien foundation in India	120	–	–
111.	Gandhi Memorial Leprosy Foundation, Hind Nagar, Wardha, Maharashtra	46	NA	NA
112.	German Leprosy Relief Association, e, Gajapathi Street, Shenoy Nagar Madras	2357	(530)	2037
113.	* H.K.N.S. Delhi	700	(300)	1700
114.	Leprosy Relief Work, Emmaus-Switzerland, 4, Gajapathy Street, Madras	1007	(449)	799
115.	The Leprosy Mission, Delhi (32 own & 37 aided centres)	3800	15787	558
		16091	39970	19095

NA Information not available.
* The figures are based on report upto March, 1986.
** Taken over by Government of Tamil Nadu.
( ) Includes both medical and social rehabilitation.

TABLE A24.4: Voluntary Organisations Training Activities under NLEP

Sl. No.	Name of voluntary organisation	No. of seats per year		Total trained till 3/87	
		Medical	Para-Medical	Medical	Para Medical
(1)	(2)	(3)	(4)	(5)	(6)
1.	Gandhi Memorial Leprosy Foundation Hindi Nagar Wardha, Maharashtra	10	78	202	2094
2.	Acworth Leprosy Hospital, Wadala Bombay, Maharashtra	—	—	353 **	497 **
3.	Bombay Leprosy Project * (MS) (German Leprosy Relief Association) Vidnyan Bhavan, II V.N. Purav Marg, Sion-Chunabhatti, Bombay (MS)	80 **	80 **	444 **	470 **
4.	Greater Calcutta Leprosy Treatment & Health Education Scheme 35/1/A, Old Bally Gunge, 1st Lane, Calcutta	—	20	—	266
5.	Leprosy Field Research Unit, Jhalda*	—	—	2	16
6.	H.K.N.S., Delhi*	4	20	200	700
7.	Holy Family hansenorium, Fathima Nagar, Tiruchirapalli, Tamil Nadu*	—	11	—	11
8.	St. Thomas Hospital & Leprosy Centre, Chettupattu Distt. North Arcot, Tamilnadu—	30	—	675	
9.	Schieffelin Leprosy Research and Training Centre, Karigiri, North Arcot Distt., Tamilnadu	20	57	554	742
10.	CHAD Hospital, Leprosy Control Programme, Christian Medical College & Hospital, Vellore, Distt. North Arcot, Tamil Nadu	—	72	—	206
11.	Hindu Mission Hospital 36, GST Road Tambaram, Madras, Tamilnadu	—	20	NA	NA
12.	German Leprosy Relief Association 4, Gajapathy Street, Shenoy Nagar, Madras, Tamil Nadu	—	99	—	89
13.	GREMALTES Referral Hospital and Leprosy Centre, 5, Gajapathy Street, Shenoy Nagar, Madras, Tamil Nadu	—	52	—	69

(Contd.)

(1)	(2)	(3)	(4)	(5)	(6)
14.	Leprosy Relief Emmaus-Switzerland, 4, Gajapathy Street, Shenoy Nagar, Madras, Tamil Nadu	–	20	–	38
15.	Hubli Hospital for the Handicapped, Hubli, Dharund, Karnataka	–	30	241 *	274
16.	Velemegna, Collekhanna, Velemegna Hospital, Karnataka*	–	16	–	–
17.	Rajendra Sevashram, Anugarah Nagar, Mairwa, Distt. Siwan, Bihar	–	45	–	710
18.	Society of Sisters of Holy Cross (St. Francis Leprosy Centre), Tanky Junction, Shretallai, Kerala*	–	120	4	322
19.	The Leprosy Mission, Delhi, and Branches at Miraj, Purulia, Salur, Naini	107	338	941	1505
	Total	221	1144	2941	8849

* Short orientation training only.

** Information up to March 1986.

TABLE A24.5: International Leprosy Organisations

	Organisation	Office in India
1.	Dr. Sunil Deepak Project Officer AMICI DI R. FOLIEREAU FOUNDATION Via Borselli 4 40135 Boiogna (Italy)	Dr. V. Ekambaram Secretary for India AMICI DI R. FOLIEREAU, Italy 23, V.P. Colony Madras-600023 (Tamil Nadu)
		Dr. Daisy Dandathil Representative in India AMICI DI R. Foliereau, Italy 2A/21, Takshila Building Mahakali Caves Road, Andheri East Bombay-400093 (Maharashtra)
2.	Mr. Hermann Kober Executive Director German Leprosy Relief Association D-8700 Wurzburg 11 Dominikanerpiatz 4 Post Fach 348 (Germany)	Mr. Jeyaraj Devadas Regional Secretary for India and Sri Lanka German Leprosy Relief Association 4, Gajapathy Street Shenoynagar Madras-600003 (Tamil Nadu)
3.	The Director LEPRA Fairfax House, Causton Road Colchoster C01 1PU Essex (U.K.)	Mr. Tilak S. Chauhan Programme Officer Lepra India, Plot No. 37 Asbestos Colony Vikrampuri, Secunderabad-500 003 (Andhra Pradesh)
4.	The Director The Leprosy Mission 80 Windmill Road, Brentford Middlesex TWS 0 QH (U.K.)	Dr. C.S. Walter Director for India The Leprosy Mission CNI Bhavan, 16 Pt. Pant Marg New Delhi-110001
5.	The Director Damien Foundation Boulevard Leopold-II, 263 1080 Brussels Belgium	Dr. N. Baktha Reddy Secretary Damien Foundation AL-189, 1st Street 12th Main Road, Annanagar (West) Madras-600040 (Tamil Nadu)

	Organisation	Office in India
6.	Dr. W. Reosenfeld President Leprosy Relief Work Emmaus-Switzerland Spitalgasse 9 3011 Bern (Switzerland)	Mr. Jayaraj Devadas Regional Secretary for India Emmaus Swiss 4, Gajapathy Street Shenoynagar Madras-600030 (Tamil Nadu)
7.	The President Sasakawa Memorial Health Foundation 3-12-12 MITA, Minato-Ku Tokyo-108 (Japan)	—
8.	DANLEP	DANLEP F-42 South Extension, Part-I New Delhi-110049
9.	UNICEF	UNICEF UNICEF House 73, Lodi Estate New Delhi-110003
10.	NORAD	Assistant Resident Representative NORAD, Norwegian Agency for Development Cooperation Royal Norwegian Embassy Chanakyapuri New Delhi-110021
11.	World Health Organisation CH-1211, Geneva 27 Switzerland	WHO, SEARO Region Indraprastha Estate New Delhi-110002

MILESTONE CHART

The broad aims of programme thrusts and design could be on the following lines:

(a) *Mass Awareness and Participation in Sixth Plan* (1982-85) — Getting leprosy accepted by the society as any other disease for which cure is available through mass education, will be the major programme thrust. The steps necessary for this purpose will include: (i) the annulment of, and amendments to the Indian Lepres Act of 1898, the Bombay Prevention of Beggary Act of 1959, and the Hindi-Muslim-Christian Marriage Acts; and similarly all Acts as referred to in Chapter IV.1*; (ii) leaders in Government and those of political parties should set an example by keeping on their personal staff those individuals who are cured of leprosy; (iii) effective use of mass media, particularly the cinema, radio and television, and incorporation of a lesson on leprosy in school manuals; (iv) mobilisation of NSS, NC and other associations of both student and non-student youth and particularly of medical colleges for spreading scientific knowledge concerning leprosy; (v) training of existing staff of the programme; (vi) strengthening the infrastructure for leprosy detection, case retention, multi-drug administration, training and rehabilitation; (vii) collection, analysis of statistical data on the performance of the programme, unit-wise, district-wise and state-wise; and (viii) effective implementation of the programme with flexibility to meet the locational specificity to fulfil the objective of the programme of eradication of the disease. It will be helpful if the Lok Sabha and Rajya Sabha and State legislatures adopt a resolution on the national resolve for the eradication of leprosy through a blend of human, economic and medical action. Health education programmes including the syllabus for medical students should be suitably restructured for promoting a greater interest and understanding of leprosy among doctors and health workers. The multi-drug regimen as per guidelines given in Chapter II* should be introduced particularly in

---

* of *Report of the Working Group on the Eradication of Leprosy*, Ministry of Health and Family Welfare, Government of India, New Delhi, February 1982.

districts where there is a high concentration of leprosy patients. A time-bound action programme with respect to the introduction of treatment schedules should be drawn up by the Union Ministry of Health and Family Welfare. Steps for the early detection of cases through mobile skin camps and other devices should be introduced. Steps should be taken to mobilise the necessary drugs through import, international assistance and through indigenous production. Every student of the MBBS course of Medical Colleges should be required to spend about 3 weeks of the internship period in a suitable leprosy hospital and detection/rehabilitation centre operated either by Government or a voluntary agency. Non-formal employment procedures involving the use of former leprosy patients should be introduced. The existing arrangements for surgical reconstruction of deformed limbs and for rehabilitation measures need considerable expansion.

In addition to steps for early case detection and cure, there is need for additional steps which can help to induce the affected patients to take the full course of treatment. Since many of the patients are extremely poor and some make a living by begging or similar methods, it is necessary to provide some assistance which would enable them to take advantage of the facilities provided for chemotherapy. The World Food Programme (WFP) has indicated an interest in supporting a project for the control and eradication of leprosy. WFP had earlier supported a project in Guyana where food was used as an incentive to attract those afflicted by leprosy to take treatment regularly in the hospital. If the outpatients attended regularly, WFP rations were issued free of charge for the patient as well as the patient's dependents, particularly children. The effect was striking in as much as most of the outpatients came regularly for treatment. A similar *Food for Leprosy Cure* project could be taken up particularly in areas where there are a large number of very poor leprosy patients. Wheat or rice, pulses, vegetable oil and milk powder could be given to the patients who attend regularly, out of commodities supplied by WFP. Another method of using WFP assistance in the integrated leprosy control programme is the use of foodgrains for a special "Food for Work" programme in a few selected slum areas with a high concentration of patients. If it can be demonstrated to the leprosy patients that their micro-environment is largely responsible for the spread of the disease, then the eradication programme can proceed faster. Thus we recommend a twin strategy for the use of commodities made available by the Government of India and WFP, viz., for case holding and for environmental improvement in areas inhabited by leprosy patients.

(b) *Attack Phase, Intensified Chemotherapy Campaign: Seventh Plan* (1985-90) — If the foregoing steps are taken during 1982-85, there should be a much wider awareness of the cause of leprosy and of the fact that it is completely curable. Social discrimination trends will then weaken. With the favourable climate thus created, it should be possible to launch a massive programme for interrupting the transmission cycle and for bringing about a significant reduction in the number of persons affected by the disease through a multi-drug treatment programme in every block where there are patients. Self-reliance in the production of necessary drugs should be aimed at to the extent feasible. The existing Sixth Plan Leprosy scheme should be implemented speedily with recruitment and training of the necessary manpower to build the infrastructure on the field and to have the population screened at least once to identify the cases in the community and to bring them under multi-drug treatment.

(c) *Consolidation Phase: Eighth and Ninth Plans* (1990-2000) — It may be possible to achieve a complete control of leprosy if an effective and safe vaccine becomes available by then. Even if a vaccine is not available, it will be possible for the few new cases developing every year to be immediately detected and treated. By the end of the century, we should then have only persons who had been affected by leprosy but who have become completely cured and rehabilitated.

PRIMARY JOURNALS

1. *Acta Leprologica* (in French)
   Editorial Office 3
   Place Claparède
   Geneva (Switzerland)

2. *China Leprosy Journal*
   (in Chinese, with summary in English)
   China Leprosy Association
   No. 2 Huifuxi Road
   Guangzhou (People's Republic of China)

3. *Indian Journal of Dermatology, Venereology and Leprology*
   Indian Association of Dermatologists
   Venereologists and Leprologists
   New D-7, Banaras Hindu University
   Varanasi, Uttar Pradesh - 220010 (India)

4. *Indian Journal of Leprosy*
   Hind Kusht Nivaran Sangh
   1, Red Cross Road
   New Delhi - 110001 (India)

5. *International Journal of Leprosy and Mycobacterial Diseases*
   International Leprosy Association
   One ALM Way, Greenville, SC 29601, (USA)

6. *Japanese Journal of Leprosy*
   (in Japanese, with summary in English)

7. *Leprosy Review*
   British Leprosy Relief Association
   Fairfax Home, Causton Road
   Colchester, Essex COI IPU (England)

8. *The Star*
   Gillis W. Long Disease Centre
   Box 325, Point Clair Br Carville
   Louisiana - 70721 (USA)

BIBLIOGRAPHY

Abe, M.; Ozawa, T.; Minagawa, F.; Yoshino, Y., 1990, Immuno-epidemiological studies on subclinical infection in leprosy, I: Clinical and immunological findings in schoolchildren and adults in Okinawa, *Nippon-Rai-Gakkai-Zasshi*, 59(2) April June, p 130-44.

Abe, M.; Ozawa, T.; Minagawa, F.; Yoshino, Y., 1990, Immuno-epidemiological studies on subclinical infection in leprosy, II: Their possible source of infection, *Nippon-Rai-Gakkai-Zasshi*, 59(3-4) July-December, p 162-8.

Abel, L.; Bonney, G.E., 1990, A time-dependent logistic hazard function for modelling variable age of onset in analysis of familial diseases, *Genet-Epidemiol.*, 7(6), p 391-407.

Abel, L.; Cua, V.V.; Oberti, J.; Lap, V.D.; Due, L.K.; Grosset, J.; Lagrange, P.H., 1990, Leprosy and BCG in southern Vietnam, *Lancet*, 335(8704) June 23, p 1536, [letter, comment].

al Kandari, S.; al Anezi, a.; Pugh, R.N.; al Qasaf, F.; al Abyad, S., 1990, Leprosy in Kuwait: An epidemiological study of new cases, *Ann-Trop-Med-Parasitol.*, 84(5) October, p 513-22.

Andersen, J.G., 1991, Amyloidosis, *Leprosy-Review*, 62(2) June, p 230, letter.

Anita, N.H.; Birdi, T.J., 1988, Leprosy vaccine: A reappraisal, *Int-J-Lepr-Other-Mycobact-Dis.*, 56(2) June, p 310-3.

Anon, 1988, WHO Expert Committee on Leprosy, *World-Health-Organ-Tech-Rep-Ser.*, 768, p 1-51.

Arain, G.M., 1991, BCG vaccination *JPMA-J-Pak-Med-Assoc.*, 41(7) July, p 150-1, [editorial].

Aytekin, A.H.; Saylan, T., 1988, Close-contact surveys and mass-screening studies for leprosy in Turkey, *Leprosy-Review*, 59(3) September, p 225-9.

Aytekin, A.H.; Saylan, T., 1988, Leprosy in Turkey, *Leprosy-Review*, 59(3) September, p 231-4.

Bagshawe, A.; de Burgh, S.; Fung, S.C.; Chuah, J.; Berry, G., 1989, The epidemiology of leprosy in a high prevalence village in Papua New Guinea, *Trans-R-Soc-trop-Med-Hyg.*, 83(1) January-February, p 121-7.

Bagshawe, A.F.; Garsia, R.J.; Baumgart, M.; Astbury, L., 1990, IgM serum antibodies to phenolic glycolipid-I and clinical leprosy: Two years' observation in a community with hyperendemic leprosy, *Int-J-Lepr-Other-Mycobact-Dis.*, 58(1) March, p 25-30.

Bagshawe, A.; Scott, G.C.; Russell, D.A.; Wigley, S.C.; Merianos, A.; Berry, G., 1989, BCG vaccination in leprosy: Final results of the trial in Karimui, Papua New Guinea, 1963-79, *Bull-World-Health-organ.*, 67(4), p 389-99.

Baker, R.J., 1990, The need for new drugs in the treatment and control of leprosy, *Int-J-Lepr-Other-Mycobact-Dis.*, 58(1) March, p 78-97.

Bastien, P., 1990, Public-health epidemiology in Vanuatu, *Med-J-Aust.*, 152(1) Janmuary 1, p 13-7.

Bechelli, L.M., 1989, Indeterminate leprosy in a population survey and in the subsequent follow-ups of children in Burma, *Acta-Leprol.*, 7(1), p 29-36.

Bechelli, L.M.; Pagnano, P.M., 1990, Reflections on some aspects of leprosy among children in Brazil and in other countries, *Acta-Leprol.*, 7(3), p 229-37.

Berhe, D.; Haimanot, R.T.; Tedla, T.; Taddesse, T., 1990, Epidemiological pattern of leprosy in Ethiopia: A review of the control programmes, *Leprosy-Review* 61(3) September, p 258-66.

Bhakti, W.S., 1988, Case detection: Are the present survey methods effective? A review of leprosy surveys in Bombay, *Leprosy-Review*, 59(3) September, p 239-44.

Bhardwaj, V.P.; Katoch, K., 1989, Detection of subclinical infection in leprosy: An 8 years follow-up study, *Indian Journal of Leprosy*, 61(4) October, p 495-502.

Bharadwaj, V.P.; Katoch, K., 1990, An overview of the current status of serological techniques in the epidemiology of leprosy, *Trop-Med-Parasitol.*, 41(3) September, p 359-60.

Bhatia, V.N., 1988, Importance of good quality skin smears to a peripheral worker in Leprosy Eradication Programme, *Indian Journal of Leprosy*, 60(2) April, p 230-4.

Bloom, B.R., 1988, The 13th Kellersberger memorial lecture, 1987: A view of vaccines against leprosy and a reflection on "appropriate science" and the Third world, *Ethiop-Med-J.*, (1) January, p 45-57.

Bloom, B.R., 1988-89, Pathogenesis of a Third World disease: Lessons from leprosy, *Harvey, Lect.*, 84, p 41-63.

Bloom, B.R.; Jacobs, W.R. Jr., 1989, New strategies for leprosy and tuberculosis and for development of bacillus Calmette-Guerin into a multivaccine vehicle, *Ann-N-Y-Acad-Sci.*, 569, p 155-73.

Borrigter, G.; Ponnighaus, J.M.; Fine, P.E., 1988, Preliminary appraisal of a WHO-recommended multiple drug regimen in pauchibacillary leprosy patients in Malawi, *Indian Journal of Leprosy Itger-Mycobact-Dis.*, 56(3) September, p 408-17.

Brightmer, M.I., 1990, New cases of leprosy in the Cross River Region, Nigeria, *Leprosy-Review,* 61(3) September, p 273-81.

Brunel, W.; Schecter, W.P.; Schecter, G., 1988, Hand deformity and sensory loss due to Hansen's disease in American Samoa, *J-Hand-Surg-Am.*, 13(2) March, p 279-83.

Cartel, J.L.; Chanteau, S.; Boutin, J.P.; Plichart, R.; Richez, P.; Roux, J.F.; Grosset, J.H., 1990, Assessment of anti-phenolic glycolipid-I IgM levels using an ELISA for detection of M. leprae infection in populations of the South Pacific Islands, *Int-J-Lepr-Other-Mycobact-Dis.*, 58(3) September, p 512-7.

Cartel, J.L.; Chanteau, S.; Boutin, J.P.; Taylor, R.; Plichart, R.; Roux, J.; Celerier, P.; Grosset, J.H., 1989, Implementation of chemoprophylaxis of leprosy in the southern Marquesas with a single dose of 25 mg per kg rifampin, *Int-J-Lepr-Other-Mycobact-Dis.*, 57(4) December, p 810-6.

Casabianca, M.N., 1990, Monitoring and evaluation of MDT programmes, *Indian Journal of Leprosy,* 62(1) January-March, p 25-32.

Chakrabarty, A.N.; Dastidar, S.G., 1989, Correlation between occurrence of leprosy and fossil fuels: Role of fossil fuel bacteria in the origin and global epidemiology of leprosy, *Indian-J-Exp-Biol.*, 27(6) June, p 483-96.

Chan, V.F., 1988, Tropical diseases of public health importance in the Philippines, *Southeast-Asian-J-Trop-Med-Public-Health.*, 19(3) September, p 361-7.

Chanteau, S.; Cartel, J.L.; Plichart, R.; Roux, J.; Bach, M.A., 1989, PLG I antigen and antibody detection in the control of leprosy in French Polynesia, *Acta-Leprol.*, 7, Supplement 1, p 128-9.

Chanteau, S.; Plichart, R.; Boutin, J.P.; Roux, J.; Cartel, J.L., 1989, Finger-prick blood collection and computer-assisted enzyme-linked immunosorbent assay for large-scale serological studies on leprosy, *Trans-R-Soc-Trop-Med-Hyg.*, 883(3) May-June, p 414-6.

Chen, P.C., 1988, Longhouse dwelling, social contact and the prevalence of leprosy and tuberculosis among native tribes of Sarawak, *Soc-Sci-Med.*, 26(10), p 1073-7.

Cho, S.N.; Kim, S.H.; Cellona, R.V.; Chan, G.P.; Fajardo, T.T.; Walsh, G.P.; Kim, J.D., 1992, Prevalence of IgM antibodies to phenolic glycolipid I among household contacts and controls in Korea and the Philippines, *Leprosy Review.*, 63(1) March, p 12-20.

Chonde, T.M., 1989, The role of bacteriological services in the National Tuberculosis and Leprosy Programme in Tanzania, *Bull-Int-Union-Tuberc-Lung--Dis.*, 64(3) September, p 37-9.

Chopra, N.K.; Agarwal, J.S.; Pandya, P.G., 1989, Impact of multidrug therapy on leprosy in Baroda district (Gujarat), *Indian Journal of Leprosy*, 61(2) April, p 179-89.

Choudhury, A.; Mistry, N.F.; Anita, N.H., 1989, Blocking of Mycobacterium leprae adherence to dissociated Schwann cells by anti-mycobacterial antibodies, *Scand-J-Immunol.*, 30(4), October, p 505-9.

Chugh, K.S.; Sakhuja, V., 1990, Glomerular diseases in the tropics, *Am, J. Nephrol*, 10(6), p 437-50, editorial.

Chum, H.J., 1989, Ten years of the National Tuberculosis/Leprosy Programme in Tanzania, *Bull-Int-Union-Tuberc-Lung-Dis.*, September, p 34-6.

Convit, J.; Sampson, C.; Zungia, M.; Smith, P.G.; Plata, J.; Silva, J.; Molina, J.; Pinardi, M.E.; Bloom, B.R.; Salgado, A., 1992, Immunoprophylactic trial with combined Mycobacterium leprae/ BCG vaccine against leprosy: Preliminary results, *Lancet*, 22, 339(8791) February, p 446-50.

Courtright, P.; Lewallen, S.; Lee, H.S., 1991, Comparison of the old and new W.H.O. leprosy disability grading scheme for occular disabilities, *Int-Ophthalmol*, 15(5) September, p 295-8.

Courttright, P.D., 1988, Defining the magnitude of ocular complications form leprosy: Problems of methodology, *Int-J-Lepr-Other-Mycobact-Dis.*, 56(4) December, p 566-73.

Crawford, C.L., 1990, In spectacular retreat, BMJ, 300(6719), p 261, letter.

Crawford, C.L., 1990, Methods of leprosy prevention, 345(6274) May 31, p 392, letter, comment.

Crook, N.; Ramasubban, R.; Samy, A.; Singh, B., 1991, An educational approach to leprosy control: An evaluation of knowledge, attitudes and practice in two poor localities in Bombay, India, *Leprosy-Review* 62(4) December, p 395-401.

Dagnew, M.B., 1989, Efficiency of leprosy control programmes, *World-Health-Forum.*, 10(3-4), p 433-4, letter.

Daumerie, D., 1991, Leprosy in the WHO African region, *World Health Statistical Quarter*, 44(1), p 16-22.

Dayal, R., 1991, Early detection of leprosy in children, *J-Trop-Pediatr.*, 37(6) December, p 310-2.

de Vries R., 1990, Old BCG replaced by new vaccine? Human leukocyte antigens (HLA) and mycobacterial disease, *Bull-Int-Union-Tuberc-Lung-Dis.*, 65(2-3) June-September, p 30-1.

de Vries, R.R.; Ottenhoff, T.H.; van Schooten, W.C., 1988, Human leukocyte antigens (HLA) and mycobacterial disease [published erratum appears in *Springer Semin Immunopathol*, 11(1), 89], *Springer-Semin-Immunopathol*, 10(4), p 305-18.

Deo, M.G., 1989, ICRC 'anti-leprosy vaccine', *Vaccine*, 7(2) April, p 92-3.

Deo, M.G.; Chaturvedi, R.M.; Kartikeyan, S., 1990, A candidate anti-leprosy vaccine from ICRC bacilli, *Trop-Med-Parasitol.*, 41(3) September, p 367-8.

Dewapur, D.R., 1989, The current state of leprosy control activities in Sri Lanka, *Leprosy-Review*, 60(1) March, p 39-44.

Dharmshaktu, N.S., 1990, Overview of leprosy problem in India and strategies of National Leprosy Eradication Programme, *Indian Journal of Leprosy*, 62(1) January-March, p 16-8.

Dharmshaktu, N.S., 1990, Progress of multi drug therapy under National Leprosy Eradication Programme, *Indian Journal of Leprosy*, 62(1) January-March, p 19-21.

Ell, S.R., 1988, Reconstructing the epidemiology of medieval leprosy: preliminary efforts with regard to Scandinavia, *Perspect-Biol-Med.*, 31(4) Summer, p 496-506.

Fadalae, A.; Ortiz, R.R., 1988, Leprosy eradication in Paraguay, *Leprosy-Review*, 59(3) September, p 267-8, letter.

Fassin, D., 1990, Influence of social perceptions of leprosy and leprosy patients on public health programmes, *Int-J-Lepr-Other-Mycobact-Dis.*, 58(1) March, 111-4.

Feenstra, P.; Tedla, T., 1988, A broader scope for leprosy control, *World-Health-Forum*, 9(1), p 53-8.

Fftyche, T., 1991, Ocular leprosy: The continuing challenge, *Int-Ophthalmol*, 15(5) September, p 289-93.

Fine, P.; Dockrell, H.; 1991, Leprosy vaccines, *Vaccine*, 9(5) May, p 291-3.

Fine, P.E., 1988, BCG vaccination against tuberculosis and leprosy, *Br-Med-Bull.*, 44(3) July, p 691-703.

Fine, P.E., 1988, Implications of genetics for the epidemiology and control of leprosy, *Philos-Trans-R-Soc-Lond-Biol.*, 321(1207) October, 31, p 365-76.

Fine, P.E., 1989, The BG story: Lessons from the past and implications for the future, *Rev-Infect-Dis.*, 11 Suppl 2 March-April, p 8353-9.

Fine, P.E., 1989, Immunological tools in leprosy control, *Int-J-Lepr-Other-Mycobact-Dis.*, 57(3) September, p 671-86.

Fine, P.E.; Ponnighaus, J.M., 1988, Leprosy in Malawi, 2: Background, design and prospects of the Karonga Prevention Trial: A leprosy vaccine trial in northern Malawi, *Trans-R-Soc-Trop-Med-Hyg.*, 82(6), p 810-7.

Fine, P.E.; Ponnighaus, J.M.; Burgess, P.; Clarkson, J.A.; Draper, C.C., 1988, Seroepidemiological studies of leprosy in northern Malawi based on an enzyme-linked immunosorbent assay using synthetic glycoconjugate antigen, *Int-J-Lepr-other-Mycobact-Dis.*, 5692) June, p 243-54.

Fine, P.E.; Rodrigues, L.C.; 1990, Modern vaccines, Mycobacterial diseases *Lancent*, 335(8696) April 28, p 1016-20, (*see* comments).

Fleischer, A.B. Jr.; Maxwell, B.A.; Baird, D.B.; Woosley, J.T.; Hansen's disease (leprosy): The North Carolina experience, *Cutis.*, 45(6) June, p 427-34.

Foster, R.L.; Sanchez, A.L.; Stuyvesant, W.; Foster, F.N.; Small, C.; Lau, Sanchez, A.L.; Stuyvesant, W.; Foster, F.N.; Small, C.; Lau, B.H., 1988, Nutrition in leprosy: A review, *Int-J-Lepr-Other-Mycobact-Dis.* 56(1) March, p 66-81.

Frankel, R.I., 1988, Hansen's disease in Hawaii: Current status, *Hawaii-Med-J.*, 47(2) February, p 48, 51-3.

Friedericks, R.C., 1991, A multi-media approach to health education, *Leprosy-Review*, 62(3) September, p 329-32.

Fytche, T., 1989, Blindness in leprosy: A forgotten complication, *Aust-N-Z-J-Ophthalmol.*, 17(3) August, p 257-60.

Ganapati, R., 1990, Leprosy control within urban primary health care, *Indian Journal of Leprosy*, 62(2) April-June, p 161-8.

Ganapati, R., 1991, Control of leprosy in India in the background of urbanization, *Indian Journal of Leprosy,* 63(3-4) July-December, p 334-41.

Ganapati, R., et al, 1989, A pilot study of three potential vaccines for leprosy in Bombay, *Int-J-Lepr-other-Mycobact-Dis.*, 57(1) March, p 33-7.

Ganju, L.; Batra, H.V.; Talwar G.P.; Mukherjee R., 1991, A rapid latex agglutination test for detection of antibodies in tuberculosis and Hansen's disease, *J-Immunoassay,* 12(4), p 579-95

Ganju, L.; Mukherjee, R.; Batra, H.V.; Talwar, G.P., 1990, Immunoblot analysis of antigens of Mycobacterium a candidate anti-leprosy vaccine using monoclonal antibodies and patient sera, *Int-J-Med-Microbiol.*, 273(3), p 378-85.

Gelber, R.H.; Murray, L.; Siu, P.; Tsang, M., 1992, Vaccination of mice with a soluble protein fraction of Mycobacterium leprae provides consistent and long-term protection against M. Leprae infection, *Infect-Immun.,* 60(5) May, p 1840-4.

Ghazi, Saidi K.; Stanford, J.L.; Stanford, C.A.; Dowlati, Y.; Farshchi, Y.; Rook, G.A.; Rees, R.J., 1989, Vaccination and skin test studies on children living in villages with differing endemicity for leprosy and tuberculosis,. *Int-J-Lepr-Other-Mycobact-Dis.*, 57(1) March, p 45-53.

Gilbody, J.S., 1991, Impact of multidrug therapy on the treatment and control of leprosy [editorial] *Int-J-Lepr-Other-Mycobact-Dis.*, 59(3) September, p 458-78.

Godal, T.; Tsega, E.; 1990, Armauer Hansen Research Institute: A 20-year old experiment, *Ethiop-Med-J.*, 28(4) October, p 203-4.

Goyder, E.C., 1988, Leprosy control in a Bombay slum: A general assessment, *Leprosy-Review*, 59(3) September, p 245-33.

Groenen, G.; Pattyn, S.R.; Ghys, P.; Tshilumba, K.; Kuykens, L.; Colston, M.J., 1990, A longitudinal study of the incidence of leprosy in a hyperendemic area in Zaire, with special reference to PGLL-antibody results: The Yalisombo Study Group, *Int-J-Lepr-Other-Mycobact-Dis.*, 58(4), p 641-50.

Gunby, P., 1992, Can leprosy be neutralized by year 2000?, *JAMA*, 267(17) May 6, p 2289, news.

Gupta, M.D.; Anantharaman, D.S., 1988, Use of soluble antigens in leprosy epidemiology, *Leprosy-Review*, 59(4) December, p 329-35.

Gupta, M.D.; Anantharaman, D.S.; Nagaraju, B.; Kannan, S.; Vallishayes, R.S.; 1990, Experiences with Mycobacterium leprae soluble antigens in a leprosy endemic population, *Leprosy-Review*, 61(2) June, p 132-44.

Gupte, M.D.; Vallishayee, R.S.; Nagaraju, B.; Ramalingam, A.; Lourdusamh, G.; Kannan, S., 1990, Inter-observer agreement and clinical diagnosis of leprosy for prophylaxis studies, *Indian Journal of Leprosy*, 62(3) July-September, p 281-95.

Hanks, J.H., 1991, Cogitations on the cultivation of Mycobacterium leprae; why bother?, *Int-J-Lepr-Other-Mycobact-Dis.*, 59(2) June, p 304-10, editorial.

Hay, R.J., 1988, The control of infective skin diseases: The lessons of leprosy research, *Br-J-Dermatol.*, 119(4) October, p 495-502.

Helber, R.H.; Rea, T.H.; Murray, L.P.; Siu, P.; Tsang, M.; Byrd, S.R., 1990, Primary dapsone-resistant Hansen's disease in California Experience with over 100 Mycobacterium leprae isolates, *Arch-Dermatol.*, 126(12) December, p 1584-6.

Holcombe, D.J., 1988, A case of leprosy in central Louisiana, *J-La-State-Med-Soc.*, 140(12) December, p 33-5.

Howerth, E.W.; Stallknecht, D.E.; Davidson, W.R.; Wentworth, E.J., 1990, Survey for leprosy in nine-branded armadillos (Dasypus novemcinctus) from the southeastern United States, *J-Wildl-Dis.*, 26(1) January, p 112-5.IAL National Workshop on "Social Sciences Research and Social Action for better Leprosy Control" 14-15 March, 1991, Karigiri, *Indian Journal of Leprosy*, 63(2) April-June, p 260-9.

Ibrahim, M.A.; Kordy, M.N.; Aiderous, A.H.; Bahnassy, A., 1990, Leprosy in Saudi Arabia, 1986-89, *Leprosy-Review*, 61(4) December, p 379-85.

Irgens, L.M.; Melo, Caeiro, F.; Lechat, M.F., 1990, Leprosy in Portugal 1946-80: Epidemiologic patterns observed ruing declining incidence rates, *Leprosy-Review*, 61(1) March, p 32-49.

Iyere, B.B., 1990, Leprosy deformities: Experience in Molai Leprosy Hospital, Maiduguri, Nigeria, *Leprosy-Review*, 61(2), p 171-9.

Jacobson, R., 1990, The face of leprosy in the United States today *Arch-Dermatol.*, 126(12) December, p 1627-30, editorial, comment.

Jagannathan, S.A., 1988, Bombay leprosy project, Report of activities: 1976-1986, *Indian Journal of Leprosy*, 60(3) July, p 473-5.

Jayaraman, K.S., 1988, Disputes delay development of leprosy vaccine for India, *Nature*, 333(6174) June 16, p 590, news

Jayaraman, K.S., 1989, Leprosy vaccine: India finally agrees to trials *Nature*, 340(6233) August 10, p 417, news.

Jesudasan, K.; Pannikar, V.; Christian, M., 1988, Infectivity of secondary dapsone-resistant cases, *Int-J-Lepr-Other-Mycobact-Dis.*, 56(3) September, p 418-21.

Jeyaseelan, L.; Rao, P.S., 1989, Determination of sample sizes for epidemiological surveys using cluster sampling technique, *Indian Journal of Leprosy*, 61(1) June, p 84-91.

Johnstone, P.A.; George, A.D.; Meyers, W.M., 1991, Occular lesions in leprosy, *Ann-Ophthalmol*, 23(8) August, p 297-303.

Kamaludin, F., 1990, Leprosy control programme in Malaysia, *Nippon-Rai-Gakkai-Zasshi.*, Jul-Dec., 59(3-4): 169-82.

Kartikeyan, S.; Chaturvedi, R.M.; Deo, M.G., 1990, The sociocultural dimension in leprosy vaccine trials, *Leprosy-Review*, 61(1) March, p 50-9.

Kato, L., 1989, Comments on leprosy vaccination, *Int-J-Lepr-Other-Mycobact-Dis.*, 57(3) September, p 693-4, letter, *see* comments.

Katoch, V.M., 1991, Recent advances in the development of techniques for diagnosis and epidemiology of leprosy, *Indian Journal of Leprosy,* 63(3-4) July-December, p 362-70.

Katoch, V.M.; Shivannavar, C.T.; Katoch, K.; Kanaujia, G.V.; Bharadwaj, V.P., 1990, Towards clinical and epidemiological application of advances in molecular biology of Mycobacterium leprae, *Trop-Med-Parasitol.*, 41(3) September, p 299-300.

Kaufmann, S.H., 1989, Leprosy and tuberculosis vaccine design, *Trop-Med-Parasitol.*, 40(3) September, p 251-7.

Kaur, I.; Kaur, S.; Sharma, V.K.; Kumar, B., 1991, Childhood leprosy in northern India, *Pediatr-Dermatol.*, 8(1) March, p 21-4.

Kaur, P.; Sharma, U.C.; Pandey, S.S.; Singh, G., 1988, Epidemiology of leprosy in tribals of Andhra plateau, *Indian Journal of Leprosy*, 60(4) October, p 577-80.

Klaassen, Witt G.M., 1989, Common diseases in Nepal, *Kans-Med.*, 90(3), p 80-1, 85.

Kohli, M.; Gangully, N.K.; Kaur, S.; Chugh, K.S.; Sharma, V.K.; Bhushnurmath, S.R., 1991, Does Convit vaccine (BCG + Mycobacterium leprae) afford protection against biochemical changes in renal brush border membrane in experimental leprosy? *Leprosy-Review*, Sep., 62(3): 269-75.

Krishnamurthy, P.; Rao, P.S.; Reddy, B.N.; Subramanian, M.; Dhandayupdapani, S.; Bhatia, V.; Neelan, P.N.; Dutta, A., 1991, Seroepidemiological study of leprosy in a highly endemic population of South India based on an ELISA using synthetic PGL-1, *Int-J-Lepr-Other-Mycobact-Dis.*, 59(3) September, p 426-31.

Kurz, X.M.; Decleracq, E.E.; Vellut, C.M., 1989, Rate and time distribution of relapses in multibacillary leprosy *Int-J-Lepr-Other-Mycobact-Dis.*, 57(3) September, p 599-606, (*see* comments).

Lancet (Periodical), 1992, Bettering BCG, *Lancet*, 22, 339(8791) February, p 462-3, editorial, comment.

Lechat, M.F., 1988, Leprosy: the long hard road, *World-Health-Forum.*, 9(1), p 69-71.

Lechat, M.F.; Decleracq, E.E.; Misson, C.B.; Vellut, C.M., 1990, Selection of MDT strategies through epidemiometric modeling, *Int-J-Lepr-Other-Mycobact-Dis.*, 58(2) June, p 296-301.

Le-Kinh-Due, 1989, Experience in leprosy control in a developing country: Vietnam, *Acta-Leprol.*, 7(1), p 69-72.

Lennon, J.L., 1988, A review of health education in leprosy, *Int-J-lepr-other-Mycobact-Dis.*, 56(4) December, p 611-8.

Leonard, G., et al, 1990, Prevalence of HIV infection among patients with leprosy in African countries and Yemen, *J-Acquir-Immune-Defic-Syndr*, 3(11), p 1109-13.

Lombardi, C., 1989, Evaluation of leprosy epidemiology in 12 countries of the Americas, 1980-1983, *Bull-Pan-am-Health-Organ.*, 23(3), p 284-94.

Lombardi, C., 1989, Hanseniasis control in Sao Paulo State, Brasil, *Hansenol-Int.*, 1989, June; 14(1) June, p 14-31.

Lord, R., et al, 1989, Skin test studies on close contacts of leprosy patients in India, *Int-J-Lepr-Other-Mycobact-Dis.*, 57(4) December, p 801-9.

Loretti, A., 1991, Leprosy control: the rationale of integration, *Leprosy-Review.*, 60(4) December, p 306-16.

Ma, H.D.; Ye, G.Y.; Shu, H.W.; Jiang, C.; Zhou, D.S., 1989, Studies on social medicine and leprosy in east China, *Proc-Chin-Acad-Med-Sci-Peking-Union-Med-Coll.*, 4(2), p 61-4.

Martineau, Needham Dominique; Lacey, S., 1991, Leprosy control activities of the International Federation of Anti-leprosy Associations, *World Health Statistical Quarter*, 44(1), p 36-46.

Mathias, T., 1989, The leprosy control programme in the People's Republic of China, *Leprosy-Review*, 60(1) March, p 62-3.

McDougall, A.C.; Georgiev, G.D., 1989, Priorities in leprosy control, *Leprosy-Review*, 60(1) March, p 1-7.

Meeran, K., 1989, Prevalence of HIV infection among patients with leprosy and tuberculosis in rural Zambia, *BMJ*, 298(6670) February 11,p 364-5.

Meyers, W.M.; Marty, A.M., 1991, Current concepts in the pathogenesis of leprosy: Clinical, pathological, immunological and chemotherapeutic aspects, *Drugs*. 41(6) June, p 832-56.

Miller, R.A., 1991, Leprosy and AIDS: A review of the literature and speculations on the impact of CD4 + lymphocyte depletion on immunity to Mycobacterium leprae, *Int-J-Lepr-Other-Mycobact-Dis.,* 59(4) December, p 639-44, editorial.

Mishra, B.; Ramu, G.; Chauhan, V.S.; Kushwaha, S.S.; Dwivedi, M.P., 1988, Leprosy deformities, II: As parameters to monitor the effectivity of leprosy control programme, *Indian Journal of Leprosy*, 60(2) April, p 260-6.

Misra, R.S., 1990, Leprosy programme in low-endemic areas of India: An assessment and suggestions for improvement, *Indian Journal of Leprosy*, 62(1) January-March, p 22-4.

Mithal, S.; Pratap, V.K.; Gupta, A., 1988, Clinico-histopathological study of the eye in leprosy, *Indian-J-Ophthalmol*, 36(3) July-September, p 135-9.

Mittal, B.N., 1991, The national leprosy eradication programme in India, *World Health Statistical Quarter*, 44(1), p 23-9.

Montreewasuwat, N.; Peerapakorn, S., 1988, Leprosy situation in Thailand, *Southeast-Asian-J-Trop-Med-Public-Health*., 19(3) September, p 515-7.

Motta, C.P.; Zuniga, M., 1990, Time trends of Hansen's disease in Brazil, *Int-J-Lepr-Other-Mycobact-Dis.* 1990, 58(3) September, p 453-61.

Mukherjee, A., 1991, Histological monitoring of vaccine trials, *Indian Journal of Leprosy,* 63(3-4) July-December, p 388-93.

Muliyil, J.; Nelson, K.E.; Diamond, E.L., 1991, Effect of BCG on the risk of leprosy in an endemic area: A case control study, *Int-J-Lepr-Other-Mycobact-Dis.*, 59(2) June, p 229-36.

Muliyil, J.; Thangavel, N., 1989, Status of multi bacillary patients "lost to follow up", *Indian Journal of Leprosy*, 61(2) April, p 229-32.

Murthy, P.K.; Subramanian, M.; Reddy, B.N.; Rao, P.S.; Neelan, P.N., 1991, A computerized information system for evaluation of

NLEP through monthly progress reports, *Indian Journal of Leprosy* 63(1) January March, p 70-7.

Naik, S.S.; Acharekar, M.Y.; Godbole, P.M., 1990, Leprosy survey in night high schools in Greater Bombay, *Indian Journal of Leprosy,* 62(1) January-March, p 116-9.

Naik, S.S.; Samant, S.G.; Godbole, P.M., 1988, Involvement of students in a leprosy health education programme: An experiment, *Leprosy-Review*, 59(3) September, p 255-8.

Nair, N.G.; Radhakrishnan, S.; Ramakrishnan, R.; Sreenivas, V., 1991, Some indices pertaining to the leprosy control programme in Tamil Nadu, based on data from a random sample of fourteen government control units, *Indian-J-Med-Res.*, 93 July, p 208-16.

Noordeen, S.K., 1988, The challenge of leprosy, *Indian Journal of Leprosy*, 60(2) April, p 149-58.

Noordeen, S.K., 1988, The present status of leprosy vaccine development, *Southeast-Asian-J-Trop-Med-Public-Health.*, 19(3) September, p 525-34.

Noordeen, S.K., 1989, Technology for leprosy control: Progress and prospects: Kellersberger memorial lecture, 1988, *Ethiop-Med-J.*, 27(3) July, p 161-80.

Noordeen, S.K., 1991, Elimination of leprosy as a public health problem, *Indian Journal of Leprosy*, 63(3-4) July-December, p 401-9.

Noordeen, S.K., 1991, Leprosy control through multidrug therapy (MDT), *Bull-World-Health-Organ.,* 69(3), p 263-9.

Noordeen, S.K., 1991, A look at world leprosy, *Leprosy-Review*, 62(1) March, p 72-86.

Noordeen, S.K., 1992, Elimination of leprosy as a public health problem [editorial], *Leprosy-Review*, 63(1) March, p 1-4.

Noordeen, S.K.; Lopez, Bravo L.; Daumerie, D., 1991, Global review of multidrug therapy (MDT) in leprosy, *World Health Statistical Quarter* 44(1), p 2-15.

Noordeen, S.K.; Lopez, Bravo, L.; Sundaresan, T.K., 1992, Estimated number of leprosy cases in the world, *Bull-World-Health-Organ,* 70(1) p 7-10.

Orege, P.A.; Obura, M.; Okelo, C.; Okuku, P.; Makokha, S.; Myawalo, J., 1990, Multidrug therapy for treatment of paucibacillary leprosy in western Kenya, Preliminary communications, *East-Afr-Med-J.*, 67(9) September, p 632-9.

Pattyn, S.R., 1991, Evolution of the leprosy problem in some African areas during the 1980-89 decade, *Ann-Soc-Belg-Med-Trop.*, 71(1) March, p 1-4, editorial.

Pattyn, S.R.; Bourland, J.; Kakeze, C., 1991, Evolution of the leprosy endemicity in Burundi during the years 1981-88. *Ann-Soc-Belg-Med-Trop.*, 71(1) Mfarch, p 57-61.

Pattyn, S.R.; Grillone, S., 1991, Leprosy in the Comores 1981-88, *Ann-Soc-Belg-Med-Trop.*, 71(1) March, p 51-5.

Pearson, M., 1988, What does distance matter? Leprosy control in West Nepal, *Soc-Sci-Med.*, 26(1), p 25-36.

Pfaltzgraff, R.E., 1990, Leprosy vaccines, *Int-J-Lepr-Other-Mycobact-Dis.*, September, p 573, letter, comment.

Ponnighaus, I.M.; Boerrigter, G.; Fine, P.E.; Ponnighaus, J.M.; Russell, J., 1990, Disabilities in leprosy patients ascertained in a total population survey in Karonga District, northern Malawi, *Leprosy-Review*, 61(4), December, p 366-74.

Ponnighaus, J.M.; Fine, P.E.; Maine, N.; Bliss, L.; Kalambo, M.; Ponnighaus, I., 1988, The Lepra Evaluation Project (LEP): An epidemiological study of leprosy in northern Malawi. II: Prevalence rates, *Leprosy-Review,* 59(2) June, p 97-112.

Ponnighaus, J.M.; Fine, P.E.; Moreno, C., 1991, Hypersensitivity to dextran in BCG vaccine, *Lancet*, 337(8748) April 27, p 1039, letter, comment.

Ponnighaus, J.M.; Fine, P.E.; Sterne, J.A.; Wilson, R.J.; Msosa, E.; Gruer, P.J.; Jenkins, P.A.; Lucas, S..B.; Liomba, N.G.; Bliss, L., 1992, Efficacy of BCG vaccine against leprosy and tuberculosis in northern Malwai, *Lancet*, 14, 339(8794) March, p 636-9.

Ponninghaus, J.M.; Mwanjasi, L.J.; Fine, P.E.; Shaw, M.A.; Turner, A.C.; Oxborrow, S.M.; Lucas, S.B.; Jenkins, P.A.; Sterne, J.A.; Bliss, L., 1991, Is HIV infection a risk factor for leprosy? *Int-J-Lepr-Other-Mycobact-Dis.*, 59(2) June, p 221-8.

Prabhavlkar, A.B.; Chacko, J.; Kharkar, R.K., 1990, Further comments on leprosy vaccination, *Int-J-Lepr-Other-Mycobact-Dis.*, 58(3) September, p 573-4, letter, comment.

Puttick, C., 1991, Leprosy in Brazil: Working at the end of the world, *Nurs-Stand.,* 9(1) January, p 10-4, (interview by Michael Gillard).

Radhakrishna, S.; Nair, N.G.; Kumar, B.K.; Jayabal, P., 1988, Implications of prior BCG vaccination programmes in Community on the protective efficacy of new antileprosy vaccines, *Indian-J-Med-Res.*, 88 August, p 197-208.

Ramanujam, K., 1989, On "childhood leprosy in Bombay", *Indian Journal of Leprosy*, 61(2) April, p 311-2, letter.

Rao, C.K.; Mittal, B.N.; Dharmshaktu, N.S., 1988, Leprosy control based on multi-drug treatment in India, *Indian Journal of Leprosy*, 60(2) April, p 290-302.

Rao, P.S.; Ekambaram, V.; Reddy, B.N.; Krishnamoorthy, P.; Kumar, S.K.; Dutta, A., 1991, Is bacteriological examination by skin smear necessary in all paucibacillary leprosy patients in mass control programmes? *Leprosy-Review*, 62(3) September, p 303-9.

Rao, P.S.; ·Kumaravelu, P.; Muthiah, B.; Durgambal, K., 1989, A study into bacteriological positivity and treatment of beggar leprosy patients, *Indian Journal of Leprosy*, 61(2) April, p 216-21.

Rao, P.S.: Sirumban, P., 1990, Screening of registered leprosy cases and its effects on prevalence rate, *Indian Journal of Leprosy*, 62(2) April-June, p 180-5.

Rapoport, B.L.; Morrison, R.C.; Sher, R.; dos Santos, L., 1990, A study of autoantibodies in chronic mycobacterial infections, *Int-J-Lepr-Other-Mycobact-Dis.*, 58(3) September, p 518-25.

Raveendranathan, O.; Nair, B.K.; Sarojini, P.A., 1991, Epidemiological significance of indeterminate leprosy: A hospital based study, *Indian Journal of Leprosy*, 63(1) January-March, p 5-11.

Rawlinson, W.D.; Basten, A., 1989, Cross-reactivity of Mycobacterium leprae and M. tuberculosis and the implications for assessment of in vitro T cell function in leprosy patients, *Trans-R-Soc-Trop-Med-Hyg.*, 83(4) July-August, p 557-9.

Ree, G.H., 1991, Pattern of leprosy in Queensland, Australia, 1855-1990, *Leprosy-Review*, 62(4) December, p 420-30.

Revankar, C.R.; Deshpande, S.S.; Pai, R.R.; Ganapati, R., 1991, Training of health posts personnel in urban leprosy programme: A preliminary report, *Indian Journal of Leprosy*, 63(1) January-March, p 97-100.

Revankar, C.R.; Goyal, N.; Sorensen, B.H., 1989, Management information system for leprosy eradication programme: An alternative information system, *Leprosy-Review*, 60(2) June, p 129-34.

Revankar, C.R.; Sorensen, B.H.; Kielstrup, R.W., 1989, Delivery of MDT through blister calendar packs in leprosy eradication programmes: A multicentre field study (phase I). Multicentre Study Group, *Leprosy-Review*, 60(2) June, p 135-8.

Richards, P., 1990, Leprosy: Myth, melodrama and mediaevalism: The FitzPatrick lecture 1989, *J-R-Coll-Physicians-Lond.*, 24(1) January, p 55-62.

Rose, P., 1989, Changes in epidemiological indices following the introduction of WHO MDT into the Guyana leprosy control programme, *Leprosy-Review*, 60(2) June, p 139-46.

Saha, K.; Rao, K.N.; Chattopadhya, D.; Lakshmi, V.; Gadi, S.; Dutta, Banik, N.D.; 1990, A study on nutrition, growth and development of a high-risk group of children of urban leprosy patients, *Eur-J-Clin-Nutr.*, 44(6) June, p 471-9.

Sampatavanich, S.; Sampoonachot, P.; Kongsuebchart, K.; Ramasoota, T.; Pinrat, U.; Mongkolwongroi, P.; Ozawa, T.; Sasaki, N.; Abe, M., 1989, Immunoepidemiological studies on subclinical infection among leprosy household contacts in Thailand, *Int-J-Lepr-Other-Mycobact-Dis.*, 57(4) December, p 752-65.

Samy, A.A.; Mancheril, J.; Manek, K.P.; McDougall, A.C., 1991, ALERT-India 1981-89: Nine years' experience of leprosy control in the slums of Bombay, *Leprosy-Review*, 62(3) September, p 315-28.

Saylan, T.; Sutlas, M.; Yuksel, A.; Cakiner, T.; Aytekin, H., 1989, The characteristics and mode of detection of the new patients encountered in the leprosy endemic province of Van within the last five years, *Indian Journal of Leprosy*, 61(2) April, p 225-8.

Sehgal, V.N.; Joginder, Leprosy in children: correlation of clinical, histopathological, bacteriological and immunological parameters, *Leprosy-Review*, 60(3) September, p 202-5, (*see* comments).

Sehgal, V.N.; Sehgal, S., 1988, Leprosy in young urban children, *Int-J-Dermatol.*, 27(2) March, p 112-4.

Sengupta, U., 1991, The utility of animal models for selection of a candidate vaccine for leprosy *Indian Journal of Leprosy*, 63(2) April-June p 153-8, editorial.

Shaw, M.A.; Turner, A.C.; Blackwell, J.M.; Fine, P.E.; Ponnighaus, J.M., 1990, Setting up HIV serology for the Karonga leprosy vaccine trial in Malawi, *Leprosy-Review*, 62(1) March, p 87-104.

Sheela, G.R.; Gopa, A.K.; Gandewar, K.L.; Ganapati, R., 1989, Multidrug therapy in multibacillary leprosy cases in an urban context — a study in Bombay, *Indian Journal of Leprosy*, 61(2) April, p 190-5.

Sheela, G.R.; Gopa, A.K.; Revankar, C.R.; Ganapati, R., 1989, Leprosy teaching in medical colleges in Bombay: A questionnaire study, *Indian Journal of Leprosy*, 61(2) April, p 233-7.

Singh, N.B.; Lowe, A.C.; Rees, R.J.; Colston, M.J., 1989, Vaccination of mice against Mycobacterium leprae infection, *Infect-Immun.*, 57(2) February, p 653-5.

Smolin, G., 1990, Hansen's disease: Have we advanced in the last 20 years? *Int-Ophthalmol-Clin.*, 30(1) Winter, p 42-5.

Soebono, H.; Klatser, P.R., 1991, A seroepidemiological study of leprosy in high- and low-endemic Indonesian villages, *Int-J-Lepr-Other-Mycobact-Dis.* 59(3) September, p 416-25.

Sreevatsa; Desikan, K.V., 1988, Evaluation of the efficacy of candidate vaccines against M. leprae infection in mice, *Indian Journal of Leprosy*, 60(2) April, p 252-9.

Stanford, J.L.; Stanford, C.A.; Ghazi, Saidi, K.; Dowlati, Y.; Weiss, S.F.; Farshchi, Y.; Madlener, F.; Rees, R.J., 1989, Vaccination and skin test studies on the children of leprosy patients [published erratum appears in *Int J Lepr Other Mycobact Dis* 57(4), December, O following 927] *Int-J-Lepr-Other-Mycobact-dis.*, 57(1), March, p 38-44.

Steenbergen, G.J., 1991, Leprosy control in Zambia, *World Health Statistical Quarter.*, 44(1), p 30-5.

Stewart, Tull D.E., 1990, Vaccines against leprosy, *Adv-Biotechnol-Processes.*, 13, 201-22.

Stitt, P.G., 1990, Chance, the prepared mind and children with Hansen"s disease, *Hawaii-Med-J.*, 49(8) August, p 309-12.

Suite, M.; Edinborough, N.B., 1989, A second report on multidrug therapy for leprosy in Trinidad and Tobago, *Leprosy-Review*, 60(4) December, p 288-99.

Sukumaran, K.D., 1988, The status of leprosy control in Malaysia, *Southeast-Asian-J-Trop-Med-Public-health.*, 19(3) September, p 519-24.

Sundar Rao, P.S.; Jesudasan, K.; Mani, K.; Christian, M., 1989, Impact of MDT on incidence rates of leprosy among household contacts. Part 1. Baseline data, *Int-J-Lepr-Other-Mycobact-Dis.*, 57(3) September, p 647-51.

Sutherland, I., 1988, Research into the control of tuberculosis and leprosy in the community, *Br-Med-Bull.*, 44(3) July, p 665-78.

Tekle, Haimanot R.; Frommel, D.; Tadesse, T.; Verdier, M.; Denis, F., 1991, A survey of HTLV-1 and HIVs in Ethiopian leprosy patients, *AIDS*, 5(1) January, p 108-10, letter.

Teterissa, M.R.; Nathin, M.A.; 1988, Leprosy control in Indonesia, *Southeast-Asian-J-Trop-Med-Public-Health.*, 19(3) September, p 511-3.

Truman, R.W.; Job, C.K.; Hastings, R.C., 1990, Antibodies to the phenolic glycolipid-1 antigen for epidemiologit investigations of enzootic leprosy in armadillos (Desypus novemcinctus), *Leprosy-Review*, 61(1) March, p 19-24.

Truman, R.W.; Kumaresan, J.A.; McDonough, C.M.; Job, C.K.; Hastings, R.C., 1991, Seasonal and spatial trends in the detectability of leprosy in wild armadillos, *Epidemiol-Infect.*, 106(3): June, p 549-60.

Ulrich, M.; Smith, P.G.; Sampson, C.; Zuniga, M.; Centeno, M.; Garcia, V.; Manrique, X.; Salgado, A.; Convit, J.; 1991, IgM antibodies to native phenolic glycolipid-I in contacts of leprosy patients in Venezuela: Epidemiological observations and a prospective study of the risk of leprosy, *Int-J-Lepr-Other-Mycobact-Dis.*, 59(3) September, p 405-15.

Valencia, L.B., 1989, Social science research on social dimensions of leprosy: Where are we going from here? *Int-J-Lepr-other-Mycobact-Dis.*, 57(4), December, p 847-63.

Van, Parijs L.G., 1990, Redefining health education in leprosy: A personal view, *Leprosy-Review*, 61(2), June, p 97-111.

Varughese, P.V.; Carter, A.O.; Wittes, R., 1989, Leprosy in Canada to 1988, *Can-Dis-Wdly-Rep.*, 15(47) November 25, p 233-8.

Venkatanarayana, B.; 1990, Eradication of leprosy, Nature. The role staff nurses can play, *Nurs-J-India.*, 81(2) February, p 41-2.

Vettom, L.; Pritze, S., 1989, Reliability of skin smear results: experiences with quality control of skin smears in different routine services in leprosy control programmes, *Leprosy-Review*, 1989, 60(3) September, p 187-96.

Virmond, M.; Duerksen, F.; Goncalves, A., 1989, Report and evaluation of Brazilian experience in the rehabilitation of patients with leprosy, *Leprosy-Review*, 60(3) September, p 214-20.

Volinn, I.J., 1989, Issues of definitions and their implications: AIDS and leprosy, Soc-Sci-Med. 29(10), p 1157-62.

Waaldijk, K., 1988, The actual leprosy situation within Katsina State, Nigeria, *Leprosy-Review*, 59(4) December, p 355, letter.

Waaldijk, K., 1989, An evaluation of 35 years of leprosy control in northern Nigeria as demonstrated in the original pilot project Katsina, *Leprosy-Review*, 60(1), March, p 59-61.

Watson, J.M., 1989, Disability control in a leprosy control programe, *Leprosy-Review*, 1989, 60(3) September, p 169-77.

Wele, D.S., 1990, Health education for the successful implementation of MDT, *Indian Journal of Leprosy*, 62(3) July-September, p 346-50.

West, B.C.; Todd, J.R.; Lary, C.H.; Blake, L.A.; Fowler, M.E.; King, J.W., 1988, Leprosy in six isolated residents of northern Louisiana: Time-clustered cases in an essentially nonendemic area, *Arch-Intern-Med.*, 148(9) September, p 1987-92.

Workshop on multidrug therapy of leprosy in low-endemic areas: An evaluation, *Indian Journal of Leprosy*, 63(1) January-March, p 132-5.

Wu, Q.X.; Li, X.Y.; Shu, H.W.; Liu, Q.; Xue, Z.Y.; Ma, Z.X.; Wei, W.H.; Ye, G.Y.; Zhu, X.E.; 1989, Evaluation of fluorescent leprosy antibody absorption test versus enzyme-linked immunosorbent assay with phenolic glycolipid 1 and their use in immuno-epidemiological studies on leprosy, *Proc-Chin-Acad-med-Sci-Peking-Union-Med-Coll.*, 4(2), p 106-11.

Yuasa, Y., 1991, MDT for all: Target oriented leprosy control program in the 1990s, *Int-J-Lepr-Other-Mycobact-Dis.*, 59(4) December, p 624-38, editorial.

Zumla, A.; James, G.D., 1989, Sarcoidosis and leprosy: An epidemiological, clinical, pathological and immunological comparison, *Sarcoidosis.*, 6(2) September, p 88-96.

INDEX